plantyou

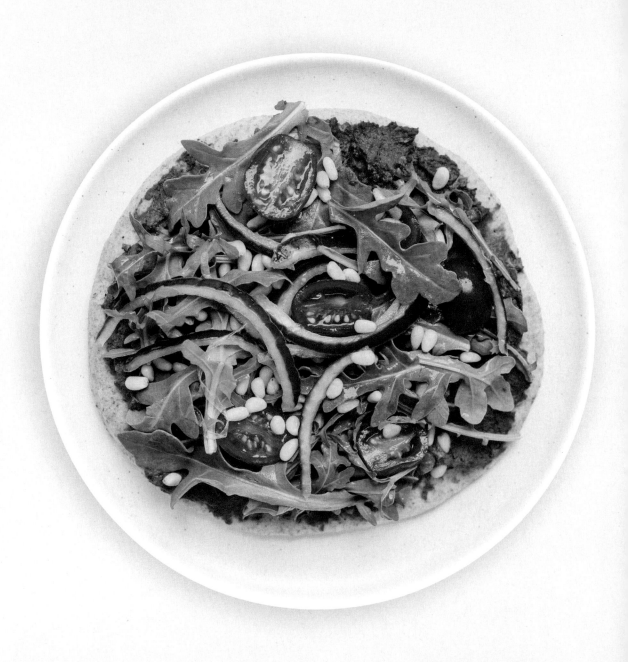

plantyou

140+ Ridiculously Easy, Amazingly Delicious
Plant-Based Oil-Free Recipes

Carleigh Bodrug

Go

hachette
BOOKS

NEW YORK

Text copyright © 2022 by Carleigh Bodrug

Food photographs copyright © 2022 by Carleigh Bodrug

Lifestyle photographs copyright © 2022 Stephanie McKnight

Cover design by Amanda Kain

Cover photograph by Sally O'Neil (@thefitfoodieblog)

Cover copyright © 2022 by Hachette Book Group, Inc.

Hachette Go, an imprint of Hachette Books

Hachette Book Group
1290 Avenue of the Americas
New York, NY 10104
HachetteGo.com
Facebook.com/HachetteGo
Instagram.com/HachetteGo

First edition: March 2022

Hachette Books is a division of Hachette Book Group, Inc.

The Hachette Go and Hachette Books name and logos are trademarks of Hachette Book Group, Inc.

The publisher is not responsible for websites (or their content) that are not owned by the publisher.

Library of Congress Cataloging-in-Publication Data

Names: Bodrug, Carleigh, author.

Title: Plant you : 140+ ridiculously easy, amazingly delicious plant-based

oil-free recipes / by Carleigh Bodrug.

Description: New York : Hachette Go, [2022] | Includes index.

Identifiers: LCCN 2021018222 | ISBN 9780306923043 (hardcover) | ISBN 9780306923050 (ebook)

Subjects: LCSH: Vegan cooking. | Cooking (Natural foods) | LCGFT: Cookbooks.

Classification: LCC TX837 .B5646 2022 | DDC 641.5/6362—dc23

LC record available at https://lccn.loc.gov/2021018222

ISBNs: 978-0-306-92304-3 (hardcover); 978-0-306-92305-0 (ebook)

Printed in China

IM

10 9 8 7 6 5 4 3

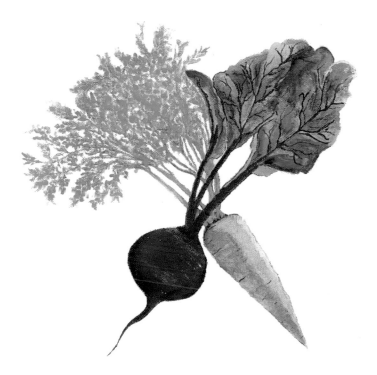

For my dad,

who survived five straight days
of recipe testing vegan, oil-free bran
muffins with me, only to have them
never make it into this book

contents

CHAPTER 1
plant-filled mornings

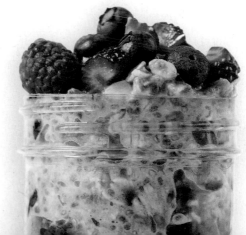

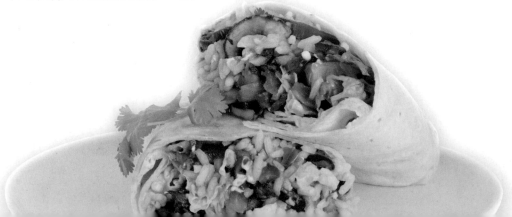

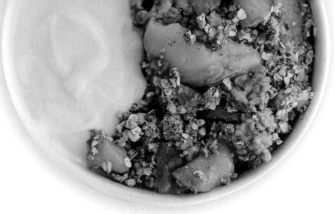

CHAPTER 5
let's get saucy

CHAPTER 6
simple sides

CHAPTER 7
plant-filled desserts

foreword

Picture yourself sitting down for a delicious dinner with your loved ones. The table is covered with a spread of mouthwatering, colorful foods—a true feast. You have everything you need to be happy...but I can level it up even more. Let's make this meal incredibly nutritious with food that heals, feeds your gut microbes, squashes inflammation, and lays out the red carpet for a long and healthy life. Food with benefits beyond just you. A way of eating that also happens to be ideal for the planet and for the animals that share it with us. A conscious approach to eating that aligns with your love for self, planet, and animals and allows you to promote health for all.

Folks, what I've just described are the joys of plant-based eating. Here are just a few of the advantages:

- **It is delicious!** All herbs and spices come from plants. There are flavor profiles from around the world for you to try. There's also tremendous variety, allowing you to mix things up and explore with your taste buds.

- **It is the optimal diet for human health.** In February 2019, the prestigious medical journal the *Lancet* published a systematic review and meta-analysis of 185 high-quality prospective studies that aggregated 135 million years of human experience into one study. Think about that for a minute...that's the entirety of human history forty-five times over. They were examining the effect of dietary fiber on human health and found that by increasing dietary fiber in our diet, we can reduce our risk for heart disease, multiple forms of cancer, and type 2 diabetes. More fiber, less problems. But where do we find this mystical salvation? Quite simply—plants. All plants contain fiber. By consuming a plant-based diet, you will get dietary fiber in spades, and simultaneously be reducing your risk of some of our most deadly illnesses. Aren't you glad you grabbed this book?

- **It is also the optimal diet for our gut microbes.** As I described in my book *Fiber Fueled*, the gut health hype is real and it's not going away. Science has shown us that our gut microbes play an important role in our digestion, immunity, metabolism, hormonal balance, mood, and brain health. The key is to feed them their preferred food—fiber! Turns out that a diverse, plant-based diet gives our gut microbes exactly what they need to thrive, and in turn helps you thrive.

- **You don't need to restrict. You can thrive on abundance.** Over the last two decades, our most popular diets have been telling us that the path to optimal health is through elimination and restriction. But we aren't any better off for it. Meanwhile, in recent years, studies have emerged showing us that there is a path through a plant-based diet that does not require us to restrict. A plant-based, oil-free diet is inherently high nutrient and high fiber. By eating this way, we can eat until we are full without counting calories, and we will accomplish our health goals and achieve a healthy weight balance in the process.

- **This isn't just about you. It's about US.** A plant-based diet is inherently conscious of the impact of our food choices on the world around us. It is impossible to ignore the disasters that have plagued our planet in recent years: unstoppable wildfires, violent hurricanes, zoonotic infections. This is about more than the world that we live in today. It's about the world that we want to leave for our children, and our children's children. Each one of us has a responsibility to do our part in trying to create a healthy planet for generations to come. Simply consuming a plant-based diet is a major step in the right direction.

Without a doubt, the benefits of a plant-based diet are powerful. But if this way of eating is a win-win-win on so many levels, why are most of us not doing it? In my experience, there are two factors that affect our motivation to transition our diet: (1) "the why," and (2) "the how."

The "why" is the accelerator that drives us. We need to know why we're going to abandon our current diet and replace it with a plant-based diet. Change is never easy! Each of us has our own story, and there are many paths that lead to a plant-based diet as the solution. My own story begins with being fifty pounds overweight, having high blood pressure, high

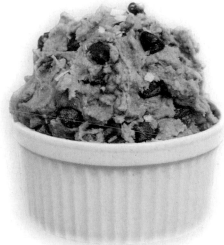

anxiety, low energy, and low self-esteem in my early thirties. Turns out that a balanced, whole food plant-based diet was exactly what I needed to thrive. For Carleigh, it began with her father being diagnosed with stage 2 colon cancer and the revelation that processed meats and red meats increase the risk for developing colon cancer. We both found our "why," and it motivated change. You have to find your own "why" and use it to fuel your desire to change to something better.

But even with all the motivation in the world, the "how" can still stand in our way. It's like a brake that slows us down, potentially even bringing us to a full stop before we reach our destination. I often see people throw up their arms and say, "Well, what am I going to eat?" My friends, this is why I am SO glad you're here. Want delicious plant-based recipes? You'll find them in these pages. Want the recipes to be simple and accessible, something anyone could do? You'll have that too. Want these recipes to be oil-free, to maximize nutrient density and allow you to balance your weight and health with abundance? Yep, we have that for you too.

Folks, a plant-based diet doesn't need to be intimidating and overwhelming. For years now I've been enjoying the easy, fuss-free recipes that Carleigh has been posting @plantyou. *Finally*, her best recipes are compiled here for an instant kitchen classic. This is the cookbook that you'll never want to put away!

In your quest to find delicious food that also promotes health, both human health and the health of the planet and the animals we share our world with, you've come to the right place. *PlantYou* is the *Ridiculously Easy, Amazingly Delicious Plant-Based Oil-Free* cookbook. I can't think of a more perfect resource for anyone looking to orient their diet toward plants, whether you're a greenhorn or a vegan veteran. Everyone wins with delicious, plant-based, oil-free meals. You bring the "why," this book will show you "how" in a fun and fuss-free way, and next thing you know, you'll be thriving on a plant-based diet and your friends will want to know your secret. You'll have to tell them that you've fallen in love with food again, thanks to your new cookbook—*PlantYou*.

Onward to health and happiness!

Will Bulsiewicz, MD, MSCI
New York Times bestselling author of *Fiber Fueled*

welcome to plantyou!

I wrote this cookbook in the midst of a global pandemic. I hope with all my heart that by the time it's in your hands, the storm has passed.

Like so many others, I grew up on a standard meat-and-potatoes diet, with steak, cold cuts, and Sunday morning bacon on weekly rotation in my family kitchen.

That all changed in 2015, when news broke from the World Health Organization that red and processed meat were now considered Group 1 and Group 2 carcinogens, with the latter ranked in the same category as tobacco smoking and asbestos.

The news was particularly rattling as my father is a stage 2 colon cancer survivor.

At the time, I was in my early twenties and thought I was eating my healthiest. Plain chicken, rice, and broccoli were on the menu every night, as I meticulously planned out my daily macros with an astronomical protein goal in pursuit of my "dream body." The reality was that my lifelong battle with constipation (to the point that I was prescribed laxatives as a kid) was worse than ever. I felt slow and groggy, and was in a constant cycle of guilt and shame whenever I'd ravenously turn to eating some of my favorite carb-filled foods, such as bread and pasta.

I'll never forget the feelings of shock, confusion, and frustration as my parents and I sat down and watched the documentary *Forks over Knives* for the first time. Everything I thought I knew about a healthy diet was flipped on its head as the veil was lifted on the propaganda surrounding the meat and dairy industries.

Armed with a degree in media theory and journalism, I began digging further into the research, reading landmark books that included *The China Study* by Dr. T. Colin Campbell and *Eat to Live* by Dr. Joel Fuhrman. The science was clear. The healthiest, cancer-protecting, and longevity-promoting approach to eating is a whole food, plant-based lifestyle (carbs and all)!

It seemed so simple. Eat more plants and lessen your risk of cancer, heart disease, and obesity, not to mention drastically reduce your environmental footprint. Why wasn't everyone shouting this from the rooftops?

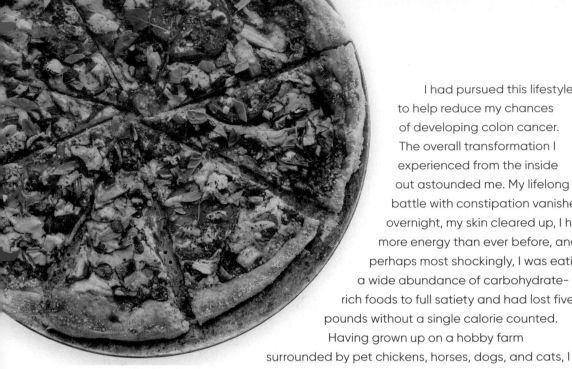

I had pursued this lifestyle to help reduce my chances of developing colon cancer. The overall transformation I experienced from the inside out astounded me. My lifelong battle with constipation vanished overnight, my skin cleared up, I had more energy than ever before, and perhaps most shockingly, I was eating a wide abundance of carbohydrate-rich foods to full satiety and had lost five pounds without a single calorie counted. Having grown up on a hobby farm surrounded by pet chickens, horses, dogs, and cats, I struggled to wrap my head around how I had separated these beloved pets from the meat on my plate for so many years. Suddenly everything was starting to click.

After going through what I can only describe as an awakening, the decision to go plant-based was a no-brainer. Figuring out what to eat for breakfast, lunch, and dinner…not so much.

At the time, I was working as a morning radio show host and news anchor in northern Ontario, Canada, in a tiny studio apartment.

Overnight, I began experimenting with plants. I noticed that most online recipes were complex, or quite frankly unappealing to someone just transitioning from a meat-and-potatoes diet. Determined to stay the course, I began cooking vegan meals by simply replacing the meat with plants in some of my favorite childhood recipes (such as the Garden Bolognese, page 140).

I felt compelled to spread the word about this amazing discovery far and wide, with benefits from reducing your environmental footprint to decreased risk of obesity, diabetes, and heart disease.

And that's how *PlantYou* was born.

It was obvious to me that there was space online for truly simple plant-based recipes. My practical, fuss-free recipe infographics quickly gained viral attention on Instagram and Facebook, and my following skyrocketed to an incredible community of over 200,000 in less than a year.

As I delved further into the literature surrounding plant-based nutrition, I noticed another consistent message from renowned plant-based doctors, including Michael Greger, Caldwell Esselstyn, Campbell, and Fuhrman. They all recommended avoiding oil in plant-based cooking, instead opting for whole food fat sources, such as avocados, nuts, and seeds. I tried my hand at oil-free cooking, and couldn't believe the impact this simple swap had on the lightness, flavor, and satisfaction of my favorite meals. You can read more on page 20 about why I've chosen not to include oil in my recipes.

In 2019, I launched my own digital meal plan program, Plant Ahead, which offered subscribers a PDF plant-based meal plan in their inbox every week. It empowered me to take the leap from my full-time corporate job to helping people eat plant-based full-time through Plant Ahead, my blog, and social channels. The program has since evolved into a weekly meal-planning web application on plantyou.com.

Over the years I have been bombarded with requests for a cookbook featuring my simple infographic recipes to help people eat more plants, and that is exactly what you have in your hands today. Thank you for empowering me to write *PlantYou*. It's a dream come true to be part of your journey.

THIS COOKBOOK HAS ONE GOAL: TO HELP YOU EAT MORE PLANTS

That one seemingly simple goal—to eat more plants—has the power to transform your life in the most beautiful, incredible way.

You see…I believe whole, plant-based foods are infinitely powerful; they contain the secret to help your body, mind, and spirit perform at their highest level.

And we're not going to get there by spiralizing zucchini, peeling chickpeas, or juicing celery.

You've got your hands on the easiest and most practical guidebook to adopting an abundant, insanely simple plant-based journey for life.

Packed with over 140 infographic recipes, featuring vegan food you'll actually want to eat (such as burgers, burritos, and big bowls of pasta to five different vegan cheese sauces), this book contains the arsenal you need to start fueling your body with nourishing plant-based foods.

THIS ISN'T A BOOK ABOUT DIETING

Actually, it's quite the opposite.

When I switched to a plant-based lifestyle, I finally discovered *food freedom*. I broke up with counting calories, limiting carbohydrates to a fist size on my plate, trying to meet a ridiculous protein quota, and scaling back serving sizes.

All along, the secret had been right in front of my nose. Simply enjoy an abundance of plant foods closest to their natural state, and reap the benefits of effortless weight maintenance, glowing skin, more regular bathroom breaks, and higher energy.

Mother Nature truly provides everything we need. In each edible plant, from baby spinach to russet potato, you will find a balance of energy, nutrients, protein, and fiber needed to fuel your body. This is without the need of synthetic protein powders, bars, meal-replacement shakes, and "skinny" teas.

WHAT IS A WHOLE FOOD, PLANT-BASED LIFESTYLE?

The term *plant-based* might conjure up images of kale salads and lentil soups, but truly that's a very small part of a satisfying and nourishing whole food, plant-based (WFPB) lifestyle.

In its simplest form, WFPB describes an approach to eating that consists of mostly or entirely foods derived from good old plants.

So, what falls under the category of a plant?

- **Veggies:**
  e.g., spinach, kale, bell peppers, lettuce, bok choy, onion, potatoes, mushrooms

- **Fruits:**
  e.g., apples, oranges, bananas, grapes, raspberries, strawberries

- **Whole grains:**
  e.g., oats, quinoa, brown rice, barley, cereals, whole-grain pasta

- **Nuts & seeds:**
  e.g., hemp seeds, peanuts, pumpkin seeds, chia seeds, walnuts, nut butters

- **Legumes:**
  e.g., chickpeas, lentils, black beans, kidney beans, split peas, tempeh

what to eat on a plant-based diet

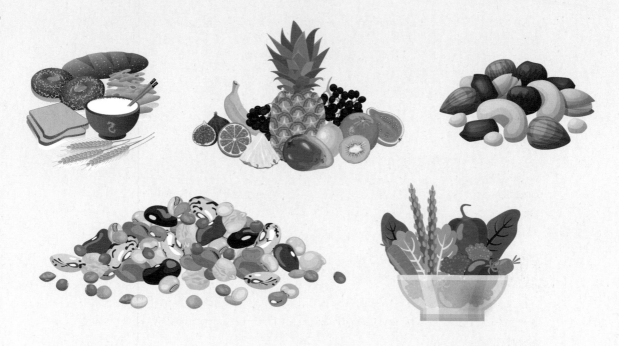

what to avoid

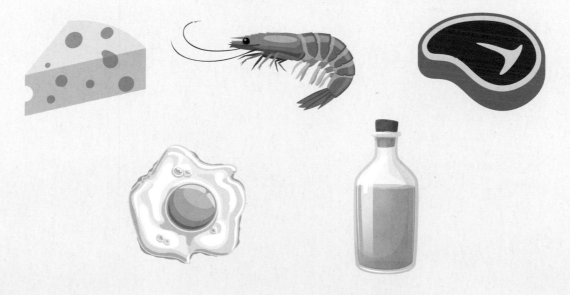

As you can see, an abundance of foods is included in the WFPB protocol. On the flip side, the lifestyle seeks to exclude animal products (including meat, dairy, and eggs), as well as added oil and refined sugar.

In this cookbook, I will equip you with tools you need to make an endless combination of taste bud–tantalizing recipes using just plant foods. Rich in naturally occurring carbohydrates, fiber, healthy fats, protein, and nutrients, these simple plant-forward recipes will have your body, brain, and soul feeling their absolute best.

Is plant-based the same as vegan?

In this cookbook, you might see me refer to both the terms *plant-based* and *vegan* when describing my recipes. The truth is, these are two very different core ideologies, and you might identify with both.

In veganism, the motivation is to avoid animal cruelty in every facet of one's life, including the clothes one wears, companies one supports, and of course the food one eats. Following this train of thought, a person could still enjoy a diet made up of mostly processed and fast foods, while still being vegan. Veganism is not a descriptor of the healthiness of one's diet.

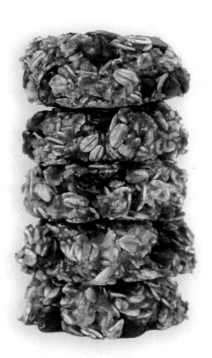

Meanwhile, the term *plant-based* originates in the health community. It describes a nourishing approach to eating, with the majority of one's diet made up of whole, unprocessed plants. This way of eating is generally pursued to achieve greater health, and does not have an ethical or moral connotation. A person who eats meat occasionally, or wears animal products, could still be consuming a plant-based diet.

Along this train of thought, a person can identify as eating a plant-based diet as well as practicing the ethical fundamentals of veganism.

At the end of the day, try not to get wrapped up in the labels. What matters is that you find your "why" for eating more plants, and use that as motivation to incrementally reduce the animal products you're consuming or using in your day-to-day life. Progress is always more important than perfection, and very few people are successful at going completely vegan overnight.

Why eat fewer animal products?

THE PLANET

Avoiding meat and dairy products is the single biggest way to reduce your environmental impact on the planet.

A study by Poore and Nemecek[1] showed that meat and dairy provide just 18 percent of calories to feed the world, yet use 85 percent of farmland. They also contribute to 60 percent of agriculture's greenhouse gas emissions.

Meanwhile, it also showed that without meat and dairy consumption, farmland could be reduced by more than 75 percent. For context, 1.5 acres of land can produce 37,000 pounds of plant-based food, but just 375 pounds of beef.

OUR HEALTH

Our health is no doubt one of the biggest drivers of the plant-based movement, and with good reason. A whole food, plant-based lifestyle may help prevent, treat, or reverse some of our leading causes of death, including heart disease, type 2 diabetes, and high blood pressure.

Research also shows that eating a more plant-centric diet can help with weight loss and weight maintenance. This is especially important as the United States grapples with an obesity epidemic, now affecting one in six children. On average vegetarians consume fewer overall calories and have a lower body mass index than do nonvegetarians.[2]

You may have also heard of the Blue Zones before, which are the five populations around the world that show the greatest longevity. On average, populations in these zones live ten years longer than the average Westerner, and include Okinawa, Japan; the Ogliastra region of Sardinia; Ikaria, Greece; Nicoya, Costa Rica; and Loma Linda, California.[3]

Researchers have identified commonalities among these populations, with one of the strongest being their plant-centric diets. Populations in the Blue Zones eat a largely plant-based diet with the majority of their calories coming from

> **Eat food, not too much, mostly plants.**
>
> **—MICHAEL POLLAN,**
> *In Defense of Food*

grains, nuts, legumes, fruits, and vegetables. They eat a very small amount of animal products consisting of approximately 5 percent of their diet.

THE ANIMALS

It is estimated that over 200 million land animals are killed for food around the world every single day.[4] In 2018, the USDA projected that each American would eat 222.2 pounds of red meat and poultry on average throughout the year.[5]

The majority of the meat, eggs, and dairy on our plates are the result of factory farming. Factory farming sees billions of animals housed for egg, dairy, and meat production. These animals are subject to extreme confinement, often injected with hormones and antibiotics for growth purposes and disease prevention, and then slaughtered at a young age.[6]

Unfortunately, it's not just animals raised for meat that are inhumanely treated. Dairy cows are artificially inseminated, then within twenty-four hours of giving birth, typically have their baby calf taken from them.[7] The cycle will continue so that the dairy cow can continue producing milk for human consumption until she is too old, and eventually sent for slaughter. Meanwhile, male calves, male chicks, and hens whose egg production has declined are all sent to the slaughterhouse as well.

There's no doubt a lifestyle that puts the focus on plants instead of animal products is an amazing choice for not only our health and our environment but also the animals we share this earth with.

BUT WHY AVOID OIL?

Before we dig into oil, I want to make it very clear that this is not an anti-fat cookbook. In fact, I absolutely love including healthy fat from whole, plant-based sources, such as nuts, seeds, and avocados, in my recipes.

With that said, I do believe oils are an overused and misunderstood product, and that there is value in learning how to cook and bake with less.

Here's why I personally prefer to avoid oil when I can, and why all the recipes in this cookbook are oil-free.

Olive oil is often touted as a healthy superfood that should be used on a daily basis in anything from

this is NOT an anti-fat cookbook.

cooking and baking to the base of salad dressings. This myth stems from the Mediterranean diet, which has been recognized as one of the healthiest eating protocols for longevity.

The truth is, it's actually the plant-forward approach to eating that has made the Mediterranean diet so successful, and not so much the oil.[8] Globally recognized plant-based physicians, including doctors Colin Campbell, Joel Furhman, Michael Greger, and Caldwell Esselstyn, all recommend avoiding oil where you can in a plant-based diet, and with good reason.

Similar to other processed foods, all oils, including olive, coconut, avocado, and canola, have had the fiber and majority of the nutrients processed from them. The result? An extremely dense source of calories and fat in a super-small serving size devoid of almost all the nutrients and fiber from the original whole food. This makes oil very easy to overconsume without dramatically changing the satiety of your meal.

Instead of using oil, the recipes in this cookbook strive to include the nutrients and fats from whole food sources, such as avocados, nuts, and seeds, leaving intact the fiber, vitamins, minerals, and antioxidants that would otherwise be stripped away.

You will find oil packed into just about all restaurant foods, processed microwave meals, chips, crackers, and more. I avoid cooking homemade meals with oil, but don't drive myself crazy trying to avoid it when I'm out to eat or at a family or friend's house.

Once you learn how to cook, bake, and make delicious sauces without oil, you'll be shocked at how easy it is!

HOW TO COOK WITHOUT OIL

Once I started cooking without oil, I never looked back! My food tastes light and intensely more flavorful without always being masked by a coating of vegetable oil. In each recipe I go over how to prepare it without oil, but here's a quick overview you can apply to just about any meal.

Sauté or Stir-Fry: Simply swap out the oil for vegetable broth or water in equal parts when sautéing or stir-frying. Sauté over low to medium heat in a stainless steel or nontoxic, nonstick pan; the temperature is important, since if you go too high, the liquid will dissipate and you risk burning your food. As you sauté such vegetables as onions, peppers, and mushrooms, they will also release their own liquids to help lubricate the pan. Add small amounts of liquid as you go, to avoid steaming the vegetables.

Baking: I opt for fruit substitutes, such as applesauce, bananas, and dates, in my baking to add a beautiful moistness to my recipes without oil. To prevent sticking, use parchment paper in your loaf and pie pans, and silicone or paper liners in your muffin tins.

Roasting: To roast vegetables, I always use parchment paper or silicone liners on my baking sheets. Before adding your vegetables or chickpeas to the oven, season well with your favorite spices, such as garlic powder, dill, and pepper, and a spritz of vegetable broth.

BUT WHAT ABOUT PROTEIN?

Over the last few decades, diet books, magazines, and online ads have made us believe that excessive protein—whether from animal products, bars, or powders—is necessary for weight loss, muscle growth, and overall health. Conversely, one of the most popular questions vegans get asked on a daily basis is WHERE DO YOU GET YOUR PROTEIN?

As Dr. Michael Greger points out on his website NutritionFacts.org:

- Adults require no more than 0.8 grams of protein per kilogram of body weight, e.g., 43 grams per day for a 120-pound female.

- On average, omnivorous Americans eat double the amount of the recommended intake.

- Even vegetarians and vegans get 70 percent more protein than they need.

- In total, 97 percent of Americans get more protein than they need, and those who don't are presumably on a calorie-restricted diet.

Every single plant, from cauliflower to lentils, contains protein, and it's where animals from cows and pigs to elephants and rhinos get theirs from as well. Eat enough calories in a day, and you will by default get enough protein, barring any unique health condition.

But what about protein combining?

You may have heard that to achieve "complete" proteins from plant-based foods, you need to meticulously combine different vegan protein sources together in meals, such as beans and rice.

Greger says this is a complete myth that spurred from a 1975 issue of *Vogue* magazine and was refuted decades ago:

> Our body maintains pools of free amino acids that can be used to do all of the complementing for us, not to mention our body's massive protein recycling program. Some 90 grams of protein are dumped into the digestive tract every day from our own body to get broken back down and reassembled, so our body can mix and match amino acids to whatever proportions we need, regardless of what we eat, making it practically impossible to even design a diet of whole plant foods that's sufficient in calories but deficient in protein.

Finally, you'll see I use tofu in many of these recipes; it is a good source of protein—and also is the source of many myths!

Soy, which is the main component of tofu, is a very misunderstood ingredient. People often believe that eating too much of it could put you at risk for breast cancer, but this is due in part to outdated animal studies. My friend Dr. Will Bulsiewicz (Dr. B) explains it best in his book *Fiber Fueled*:

> There's been some debate about soy due to the perception of it carrying estrogen, but I want you to understand that phytoestrogens aren't estrogen, nor do they act like human estrogen. Instead, phytoestrogens are isoflavones, one of the unique phytochemicals in soy beans…They have a number of unique health benefits, including: lowering cholesterol, strengthening bones, treating menopausal symptoms, lowering risk of coronary heart disease, and reducing risk of prostate/colon/breast/ovarian cancers.

Dr. B recommends purchasing only non-GMO and organic soy products, such as tofu, miso, tempeh, and tamari. Tempeh is fermented tofu with a chewier consistency and a nutty, earthy flavor. Some people don't like the taste or texture of tofu, but I think that's just because they don't know how to cook it to maximize its deliciousness. See page 52 for basic preparation tips.

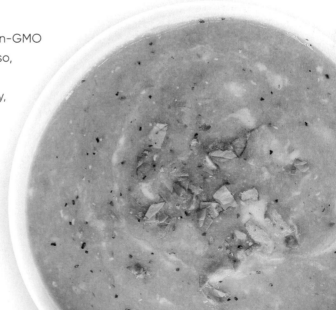

GET FIBER FUELED!

Dr. B's focus on fiber is something we should all be aware of. While everyone is so wrapped up in protein, less than 3 percent of Americans get the recommended daily intake of fiber, which is vital for gut health, cancer prevention, and weight loss. The best way to increase the amount of fiber you're eating? Include a large diversity and abundance of whole, plant-based foods in your diet. For this, we've got you covered!

A WORD ABOUT NUTRITION

I'm a big believer in counting plants instead of calories. I encourage you to let go of meticulously calculating macronutrient information and instead focus on increasing the nutrient density of your meals by fueling your body with whole, unprocessed foods as showcased in these recipes. In my opinion, one of the biggest benefits of a plant-based lifestyle is that you can enjoy an abundance of whole, unprocessed foods until you're full, without needing to track each bite.

Instead of including the nutritional estimates with each recipe, I have placed these figures at the back as a courtesy for your convenience if you would like to see them.

Nutrition information can vary massively for a recipe based on the precision of measurements, ingredients, and brands used, freshness of produce, or the source of the nutrition data. If you are using this information for anything other than curiosity, please make your own calculations based on actual ingredients used in your recipe, to ensure accuracy. For example, one brand of almond milk might have 30 calories per cup, and another 100. When in doubt, opt for such ingredients with no added sugar or preservatives.

When referring to such ingredients as rolled oats or soy milk, I am referring to a gluten- and nut-free version of that ingredient, whether noted or not. You are responsible for ensuring that each ingredient meets your dietary requirements, whether they need to be gluten-, nut-, or soy-free for your health and safety.

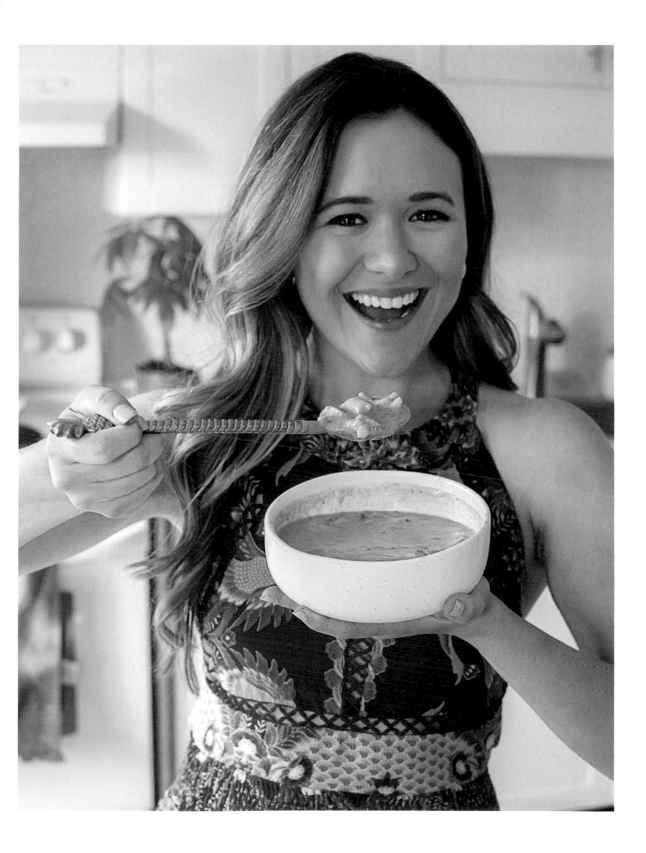

SAMPLE SHOPPING LIST

If you're new to a plant-based lifestyle, your grocery trips may look a little different from what you're used to. We put a big focus on fresh produce, and you'll probably find yourself focused on the outer edges of the grocery store. It's time to embrace new flavors, ingredients, and cuisines! I've compiled a sample shopping list with ingredients I use on a weekly basis, to get you started.

I also recommend checking out an international or Asian grocery store if you have one locally. They usually have a greater variety of fresh produce, and the prices are typically more reasonable.

This shopping list is pretty extensive, so don't be afraid to pick up just the ingredients in the recipes you'd like to try first. You can build up your pantry over time!

Important note: This cookbook is designed for simplicity and convenience. In all cases, plant milks can be homemade, canned tomatoes can be hand crushed or diced, and beans can be cooked ahead of time from scratch and substituted one for one according to measurements. Strive to purchase canned goods BPA-free, with little to no added sodium or sugar.

VEGETABLES

Keep in mind, this is a list of vegetables I use most frequently in my recipes. Feel free to go nuts in the fruit and vegetable aisles of your grocery store and experiment with different ingredients!

Arugula

Avocados

Beets

Bell peppers

Broccoli

Broccoli sprouts

Carrots

Cauliflower

Celery

Cremini mushrooms

Cucumber

Garlic

Green beans

Kale

Onions (red, yellow, Spanish, etc.)

Parsley

Portobello mushrooms

Potatoes (Yukon Gold, russet, sweet, etc.)

Radishes

Romaine lettuce

Spinach

Squash

Tomatoes

Zucchini

FRUITS

Apples

Bananas

Blueberries

Lemons

Mangoes

Medjool dates

Oranges

Pineapple

Raspberries

Strawberries

Watermelon

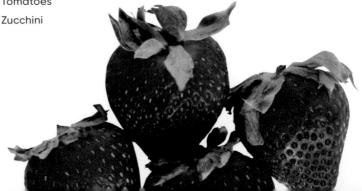

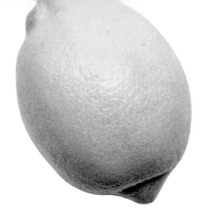

PANTRY

Note: Strive to purchase canned goods BPA-free, with little to no added sodium or sugar.

Beans, canned or dried (black, chickpeas, kidney, navy, pinto, etc.)

Lentils, canned or dried (brown, green, red, etc.)

Coconut milk, low-fat if desired

Cornstarch or arrowroot powder

Jackfruit, canned, in brine or water, no syrup

Pasta sauce (check for dairy, low sodium, sugar, and added oils)

Pure pumpkin puree (not pumpkin pie filling)

Quinoa

Rice (brown, basmati, or jasmine)

Rolled oats

Tomato paste

Tomatoes crushed, canned, jarred, or cartons

Vegan sourdough or sprouted-grain bread

Whole-grain or gluten-free flour

Whole-grain, brown rice pasta, chickpea pasta, red lentil pasta, etc.

Whole-grain or corn tortillas

NUTS & SEEDS

Purchase nuts and seeds without the addition of salt and oil when possible.

Almonds

Cashews

Walnuts

Almond butter, unsweetened

Peanut butter, unsweetened

Tahini

Chia seeds

Flaxseeds (you can purchase whole or ground; you will want to grind for using)

Hemp hearts (also known as hemp seeds)

Pumpkin seeds

REFRIGERATOR

Plant milks: unsweetened almond, cashew, soy, or oat (Can also be purchased shelf-stable)

Tempeh

Tofu, extra-firm and soft

SPICES

Black pepper

Chili powder

Cinnamon

Cumin

Curry powder

Garam masala

Garlic powder

Ginger

Italian seasoning

Nutritional yeast

Onion powder

Oregano

Paprika

Sea salt

Thyme

Turmeric

CONDIMENTS

Balsamic vinegar

Cider vinegar

Hot sauce

Ketchup, low-sugar

Pure maple syrup

Red wine vinegar

Soy sauce, tamari, or coconut aminos

Vegetable broth or vegan bouillon

BAKING

Baking powder

Baking soda

Oat flour, whole wheat flour, buckwheat flour, spelt flour etc.

Pure vanilla extract

Unsweetened applesauce

Vegan dark chocolate chips

FREEZER

Green peas

Mixed berries

Vegetable medley

COOKING EQUIPMENT

You don't need a heck of a lot of fancy cooking utensils to whip up the majority of these recipes. Here is a list of the basics I use on a daily basis that I would recommend having in your kitchen arsenal.

APPLIANCES

Essentials

Blender (high-speed, such as Vitamix or Ninja, if possible)

Food processor

Nice to have

Instant Pot

Slow cooker

Air fryer

Immersion blender

COOKWARE AND BAKEWARE

Baking sheet (13 x 18-inch recommended)

Large stockpot with lid or Dutch oven (5- to 12-quart recommended)

Medium-size saucepan with lid

Large nonstick or stainless steel skillet with lid (10- to 12-inch recommended)

Muffin tin (standard 12-well recommended)

Loaf pan (standard 8½ x 4½-inch recommended)

Parchment paper or silicone baking sheets

BASIC UTENSILS

Cutting board

Chef's knife

Paring knife

Measuring cups

Measuring spoons

Mixing bowls

Slotted spoon

Spatula

Tongs

STORAGE CONTAINERS

Lidded glass or BPA-free plastic containers

Mason jars (8-ounce for overnight oats, 16-ounce for smoothies, 32-ounce for storing broth)

Reusable freezer bags

BASIC COOKING AND PREP TIPS

Here is a basic cooking chart for my frequently used grains, beans, and starches. You will often find that I recommend canned beans in my recipes, and this is simply to make life easy. If you'd prefer to cook them from scratch, this chart is a great guide.

How to use this chart: Rinse the grains or legumes in a fine-mesh sieve before cooking to help remove debris. Place in water or vegetable broth and bring to a boil. Lower the heat and simmer for the suggested amount of time.

1 cup (250 ml) grain or legume or starch	Water needed	Cooking time and notes	Cups yielded
Black beans	3 cups (710 ml)	Soak overnight, drain and rinse, then simmer for 1¼ hours.	2¼ cups (530 ml)
Chickpeas	3 cups (710 ml)	Soak overnight, drain and rinse, then simmer for 1¼ hours.	2 cups (475 ml)
Kidney beans	3 cups (710 ml)	Soak overnight, drain and rinse, then simmer for 1 hour.	2¼ cups (530 ml)
Navy beans	3 cups (710 ml)	Soak overnight, drain and rinse, then simmer for 1¼ hours.	2¾ cups (650 ml)
Pinto beans	3 cups (710 ml)	Soak overnight, drain and rinse, then simmer for 1¼ hours.	2¾ cups (650 ml)
Green or brown lentils	3 cups (710 ml)	Rinse. Cook for 30 minutes, drain excess water after cooking.	2½ cups (591 ml)
Red lentils	2 cups (250 ml)	Rinse. Cook for 15 to 20 minutes, drain excess water after cooking.	2½ cups (591 ml)
Quinoa	2 cups (475 ml)	Rinse. Cook for 20 minutes, plus 5 minutes of steaming.	2¾ cups (650 ml)
Brown rice	2 cups (475 ml)	55 minutes	3 cups (710 ml)
Basmati rice	1¾ cups (415 ml)	35 minutes	3 cups (710 ml)
Wild rice	2½ cups (590 ml)	50 minutes	4 cups (945 ml)

How to Press Tofu

Most recipes using extra-firm tofu call for it to be pressed. Pressing tofu simply means that some of the water is being squeezed out of it to obtain a firmer, heartier consistency. To press your tofu:

1. Place a cutting board on your kitchen counter.

2. Wrap the tofu in a clean cloth or paper towel and set something heavy on top of it, for instance, a ceramic cooking pot, or another cutting board with something heavy, such as a few books, stacked on top. Allow the tofu to be pressed for 15 minutes to an hour, depending on your preference. If you find you are preparing tofu often, you can also purchase a tofu press for a reasonable price online or in kitchenware stores.

MAKE YOUR LIFE EASIER WITH BATCH COOKING

Whenever someone is transitioning to a plant-based lifestyle, I always recommend trying out batch cooking or meal prepping. By setting aside a few hours at the beginning of the workweek, usually on Sunday, you can massively cut down on your cooking and cleaning during busy nights. This will also set you up for success by having healthy meals or snacks prepared ahead of time.

You can approach this by either cooking complete meals, or preparing separate ingredients, such as quinoa and chopped vegetables, ahead of time, which then can become part of several different meals.

Most important, before you head out to the grocery store, create a rough meal plan and schedule for you and/or your family, and then prep an ingredients/shopping list. This will ensure you only pick up what you need for the week, lowering your grocery bill and reducing food waste.

If you are looking for meal prep–friendly recipes that can last a few days in the fridge and reheat well, I would definitely recommend any of our overnight oats on pages 34–39, and soup recipes on pages 76–101.

TIPS BEFORE WE GET STARTED

If you're brand-new to a plant-based lifestyle, I have some tips to make the transition a whole lot easier. First of all, please know that this is a judgment-free zone! Eating plant-based meals 70 to 80 percent of the time at the start is more important than trying to overhaul your entire diet overnight and quitting because it wasn't sustainable.

Here are some simple yet effective ways to ease yourself in:

- If you are eating meat, start treating it as a side dish rather than the main portion of your meal. This will make it easier to start seeing how dishes can shine without meat, while also allowing flexibility if you are the only person in your family transitioning.

- Look at your favorite cuisines and think about how you can swap out the animal products in the dish for plant-based alternatives. For example, replace the ground beef in your Bolognese pasta sauce with lentils instead. This maintains familiarity in your diet, while also moving toward more plant-based meals.

- Serve a large salad or soup before you eat your main meal of the day.

- Rather than relying on processed vegan foods, such as "vegan chicken fingers" or "vegan cheeses," try focusing on whole, unrefined foods. Check out Chapter 5 to see some of my favorite homemade vegan salad dressings and cheese sauces.

- Find your "why" for going plant-based. Maybe it's your health, the planet, or the animals. I would highly recommend watching the documentaries *Game Changers*, *What the Health*, and *Food Choices* on Netflix. If you prefer to read, *Fiber Fueled*, *How Not to Die*, *The China Study*, and *Eat to Live* are all excellent.

- Follow me on Instagram (@plantyou), or subscribe to my weekly meal plan app at plantyou.com! We have a whole judgment-free community of plant-based foodies to help you in your journey.

Envision this cookbook as your secret weapon to fueling your body with more plants than ever before. I've covered all the bases, providing ridiculously easy and insanely delicious plant-based meals for breakfast, lunch, dinner, and dessert.

Every great cookbook has an image with its recipes to show the reader exactly what they're making. With *PlantYou*, I have taken this one step further, providing infographics that demonstrate the core ingredients that go into preparing each meal. The goal is to make every step, from the menu planning and grocery shopping to cooking, as effortless as possible.

I encourage you to read the entire recipe before beginning. Don't skip the headnotes! They include some helpful tips and tricks to get you started.

Most of all, have fun with it and make these recipes your own. Almost any vegetable in my recipes can be swapped for another, and meals made gluten-free as needed. The meals in this cookbook are simple and straightforward so that they can be customized to your individual tastes and desires, empowering you to adopt plant-based eating for life.

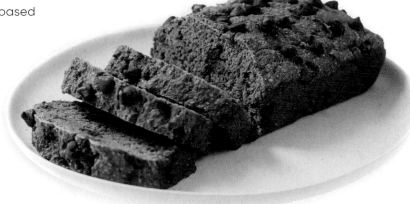

plant-filled mornings

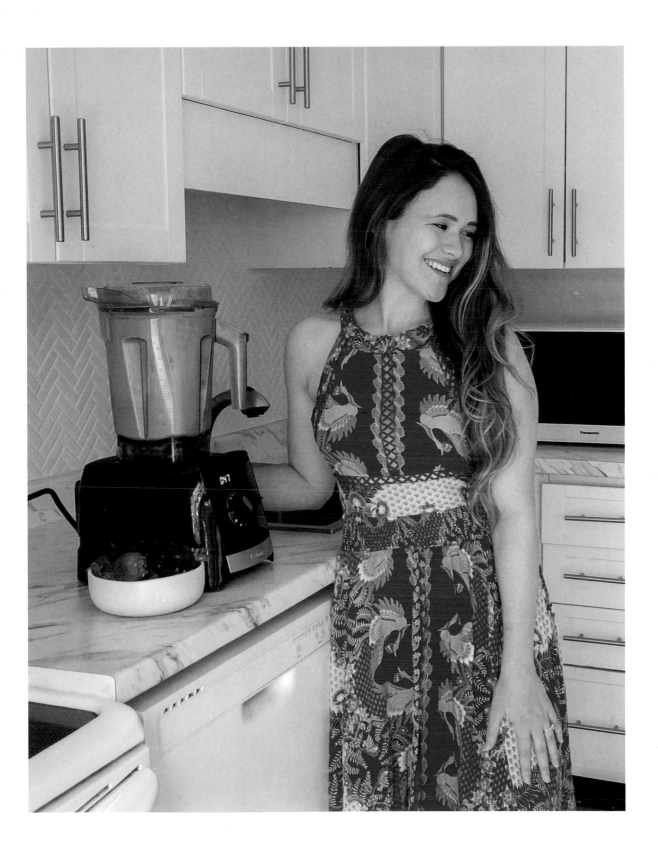

overnight oats & breakfast puddings

Overnight oats are a delicious breakfast you can prepare in advance and enjoy all week long. They also happen to be great for you, boasting a powerful trifecta of fiber, protein, and energy to start your morning on the right foot. It's no surprise that renowned plant-based doctors Joel Fuhrman and Michael Greger both like to start their day with oats.

Just in case oats don't strike your fancy, I've also included a few breakfast puddings, packed with fiber, nutrients, and plant-based deliciousness you're sure to love.

In any of these recipes, unsweetened almond milk can be replaced with cashew milk, oat milk, or soy milk as desired.

For a nut-free version, use soy or oat milk, and omit the walnuts.

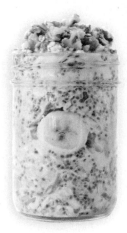
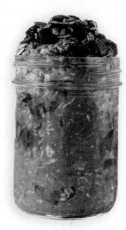
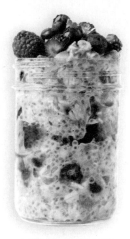
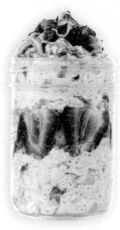

banana walnut explosion
page 36

midnight chocolate cherry
page 36

antioxidant oat cups
page 37

pb & jelly
page 37

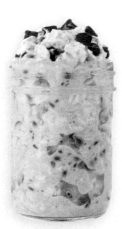
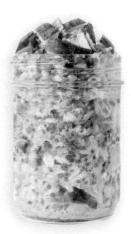
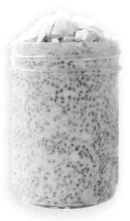
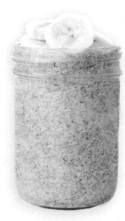

chocolate chip cookie dough
page 38

granny's apple pie
page 38

coo-coo for coconuts chia pudding
page 39

flaxmeal pudding
page 39

banana walnut explosion

MAKES 1 serving ✦ **FROM START TO FINISH:** 5 minutes (refrigerate overnight)

½ cup rolled oats

¾ cup unsweetened almond milk

2 teaspoons chia seeds

½ banana, mashed

½ teaspoon ground cinnamon, Ceylon if possible

1 tablespoon chopped walnuts, for topping

Simply combine all the ingredients in a bowl, and refrigerate in a jar or sealable container overnight to thicken.

ROLLED OATS   ALMOND MILK   CHIA SEEDS   BANANA   CINNAMON   WALNUTS

midnight chocolate cherry

MAKES 1 serving ✦ **FROM START TO FINISH:** 5 minutes (refrigerate overnight)

½ cup rolled oats

¾ cup unsweetened almond milk

2 teaspoons chia seeds

2 tablespoons unsweetened cocoa powder

¼ cup pitted and chopped cherries

1 tablespoon vegan dark chocolate chips

1 tablespoon pure maple syrup

Simply combine all the ingredients in a bowl, and refrigerate in a jar or sealable container overnight to thicken.

ROLLED
OATS   ALMOND
MILK   CHIA SEEDS   COCOA
POWDER   CHERRIES   DARK
CHOCOLATE
CHIPS   MAPLE
SYRUP

antioxidant oat cups

MAKES 1 serving ✦ **FROM START TO FINISH:** 5 minutes (refrigerate overnight)

½ cup rolled oats

¾ cup unsweetened cashew milk

½ cup fresh mixed berries, crushed

2 teaspoons chia seeds

½ teaspoon pure vanilla extract

Simply combine all the ingredients in a bowl, and refrigerate in a jar or sealable container overnight to thicken.

ROLLED OATS   CASHEW MILK   FRESH MIXED BERRIES   CHIA SEEDS   VANILLA EXTRACT

pb & jelly

MAKES 1 serving ✦ **FROM START TO FINISH:** 5 minutes (refrigerate overnight)

½ cup rolled oats

¾ cup unsweetened almond milk

4 strawberries, hulled and diced

2 teaspoons natural peanut butter

2 teaspoons chia seeds

1 teaspoon pure maple syrup

Simply combine all the ingredients in a bowl, and refrigerate in a jar or sealable container overnight to thicken.

ROLLED OATS   ALMOND MILK   STRAWBERRIES   PEANUT BUTTER   CHIA SEEDS   MAPLE SYRUP

 note For a peanut-free version, use tahini instead of peanut butter.

chocolate chip cookie dough

MAKES 1 serving ✦ **FROM START TO FINISH:** 5 minutes (refrigerate overnight)

½ cup rolled oats

½ cup unsweetened cashew milk

¼ cup unsweetened coconut yogurt

1 tablespoon pure maple syrup

1 tablespoon vegan dark chocolate chips

½ teaspoon pure vanilla extract

¼ teaspoon ground cinnamon, Ceylon if possible

Simply combine all the ingredients in a bowl, and refrigerate in a jar or sealable container overnight to thicken.

| ROLLED OATS | CASHEW MILK | COCONUT YOGURT | MAPLE SYRUP | DARK CHOCOLATE CHIPS | VANILLA EXTRACT | CINNAMON |

granny's apple pie

MAKES 1 serving ✦ **FROM START TO FINISH:** 5 minutes (refrigerate overnight)

1 apple, Granny Smith if possible, cored, peeled, and grated

½ cup rolled oats

¾ cup unsweetened almond milk

1 tablespoon pure maple syrup

2 teaspoons chia seeds

½ teaspoon ground cinnamon, Ceylon if possible

Simply combine all the ingredients in a bowl, and refrigerate in a jar or sealable container overnight to thicken.

| APPLE | ROLLED OATS | ALMOND MILK | MAPLE SYRUP | CHIA SEEDS | CINNAMON |

coo-coo for coconuts
chia pudding

MAKES 1 serving ✦ **FROM START TO FINISH:** 5 minutes (refrigerate overnight)

½ cup unsweetened coconut yogurt

½ cup unsweetened almond milk

¼ cup chia seeds

½ teaspoon pure vanilla extract

Simply combine all the ingredients in a bowl, and refrigerate in a jar or sealable container overnight to thicken.

COCONUT YOGURT

ALMOND MILK

CHIA SEEDS

VANILLA EXTRACT

flaxmeal pudding

MAKES 1 serving ✦ **FROM START TO FINISH:** 5 minutes (refrigerate overnight)

¼ cup ground flaxseeds

⅓ cup unsweetened almond milk

1 banana, mashed

1 teaspoon pure maple syrup

½ teaspoon ground cinnamon, Ceylon if possible

Simply combine all the ingredients in a bowl, and refrigerate in a jar or sealable container overnight to thicken.

GROUND FLAXSEEDS

ALMOND MILK

BANANA

MAPLE SYRUP

CINNAMON

banana stovetop oats

I love this oatmeal on a cool fall morning, topped with a generous sprinkle of cinnamon. The bananas provide a natural sweetness, so you don't need any added sugar. This recipe is also delicious with sautéed apples or peaches instead of banana.

MAKES 1 serving ✦ **FROM START TO FINISH:** 10 minutes

1 banana

1 cup unsweetened cashew milk

½ cup rolled oats

½ teaspoon cinnamon, Ceylon if possible, plus more for topping (optional)

½ teaspoon chia seeds

Walnuts, for topping (optional)

1. Combine all the ingredients, except the walnuts, in a pot over medium heat.

2. With a fork, mash the banana in the pot and mix the ingredients until combined.

3. Cook until thickened, stirring constantly, for about 8 minutes. Serve topped with more cinnamon and walnuts as desired.

note For a nut-free version, use oat or soy milk, and omit the walnuts.

BANANA

CASHEW MILK

ROLLED OATS

CINNAMON

CHIA SEEDS

WALNUTS (OPTIONAL)

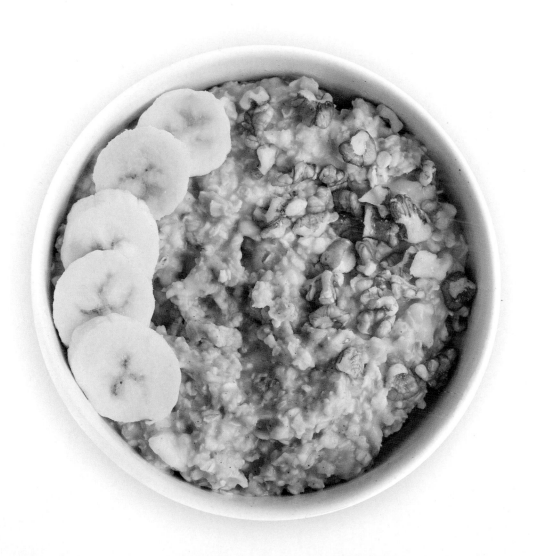

plant-filled mornings

superseed muesli

You know those hot sauce commercials that have a sweet old lady saying, "I put that sh*t on everything"? That's how I feel about this muesli. It's amazing sprinkled on oatmeal, cereal, vegan yogurt, nice cream, or even your morning smoothie. If you're looking to punch up your intake of essential omega-3 and omega-6 fatty acids, fiber, and antioxidants, whip up a fresh batch of this Superseed Muesli each week.

MAKES 12 servings ✦ **FROM START TO FINISH:** 20 minutes

3 cups rolled oats

½ cup coconut flakes

½ cup dried cranberries

⅓ cup ground flaxseeds

⅓ cup cacao nibs

⅓ cup chia seeds

¼ cup pumpkin seeds

1. Preheat the oven to 350°F and line a baking sheet with parchment paper. Spread the oats on the baking sheet and cook for 10 minutes.

2. Allow to cool to room temperature and combine with all the other ingredients in a large bowl until mixed thoroughly.

3. Store in a sealed container in a dry pantry for up to 1 month.

ROLLED OATS

COCONUT FLAKES

DRIED CRANBERRIES

GROUND FLAXSEEDS

CACAO NIBS

CHIA SEEDS

PUMPKIN SEEDS

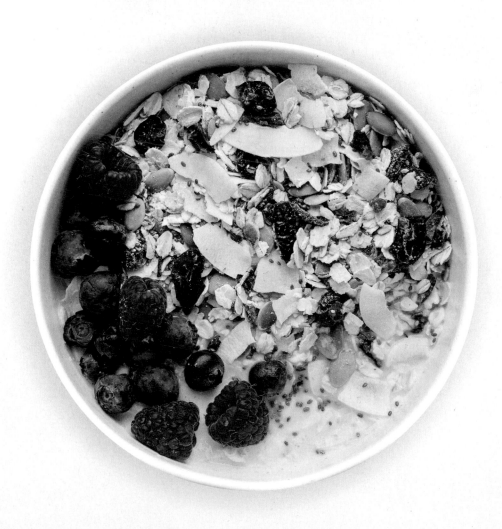

plant-filled mornings

bravocado toast

Let me introduce you to the last avocado toast recipe you'll ever need! Creamy mashed avocado is generously spread over toasted sourdough bread, topped with a hint of lemon juice, and a pinch of flaky salt, and finished off with a slightly bitter note of broccoli sprouts. Not only is avocado just delicious, you'll be happy to know it's also an excellent source of healthy fats, dietary fiber, and vitamin C.

MAKES 1 serving ✦ **FROM START TO FINISH:** 5 minutes

½ ripe avocado, pitted and peeled

½ teaspoon freshly squeezed lemon juice

1 slice vegan sourdough bread, toasted

½ teaspoon hemp hearts

½ teaspoon red pepper flakes

Pinch of flaky salt

¼ cup broccoli sprouts (optional; replace with any preferred sprout as desired)

1. Mash the avocado in a bowl along with the lemon juice.

2. Spread on top of the sourdough bread with a fork, and sprinkle with the hemp hearts, red pepper flakes, and flaky salt. Finish by topping with broccoli sprouts, if desired.

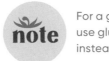

note

For a gluten-free version, use gluten-free sourdough instead.

AVOCADO

LEMON

VEGAN
SOURDOUGH
BREAD

HEMP HEARTS

RED PEPPER
FLAKES

FLAKY SALT

BROCCOLI
SPROUTS
(OPTIONAL)

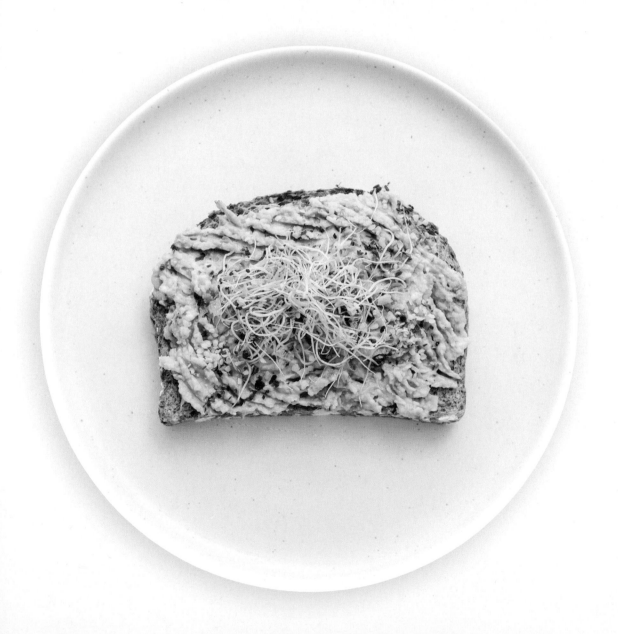

sunshine scramble

A tofu scramble completelyreplaced my desire for scrambled eggs. When it's cooked right, you'd be hard-pressed to tell the difference between the two, with the tofu scramble boasting an amazing 24 grams of protein per serving! The biggest game changer you can make to your tofu scramble is getting hold of some black salt. This salt, also known as *kala namak* or Himalayan black salt, is sourced from India and tastes surprisingly like egg because of the high sulfur content. You can find this salt at most natural food stores or online.

MAKES 2 servings ✦ **FROM START TO FINISH:** 12 minutes

½ yellow onion, diced

1 (16-ounce) package extra-firm tofu

½ tomato, chopped

½ teaspoon black salt (kala namak) (optional)

¼ teaspoon ground turmeric

¼ teaspoon garlic powder

1 teaspoon nutritional yeast (optional)

1 handful of spinach or fresh parsley

1. Combine the onion with 1 to 2 tablespoons of water in a nonstick skillet over medium heat.

2. While the onion softens, place the tofu on a plate or cutting board and mash it with the back of a fork into bite-size pieces.

3. Add the tofu to the skillet. Next, add the chopped tomato, black salt (if using), turmeric, garlic powder, and nutritional yeast (if using), and stir with a spatula to combine.

4. Sauté for 5 to 8 minutes over medium heat, or until the tofu has softened and the tomato has cooked. One minute before removing from the heat, add the spinach and stir around until wilted.

5. Enjoy with salsa (pages 216–219), vegan toast, Cowboy Casanova Breakfast Hash (page 50), or Tempeh Bacon (page 52).

YELLOW ONION

EXTRA-FIRM TOFU

TOMATO

**KALA NAMAK (BLACK SALT)
(OPTIONAL)**

TURMERIC

GARLIC POWDER

**NUTRITIONAL YEAST
(OPTIONAL)**

SPINACH

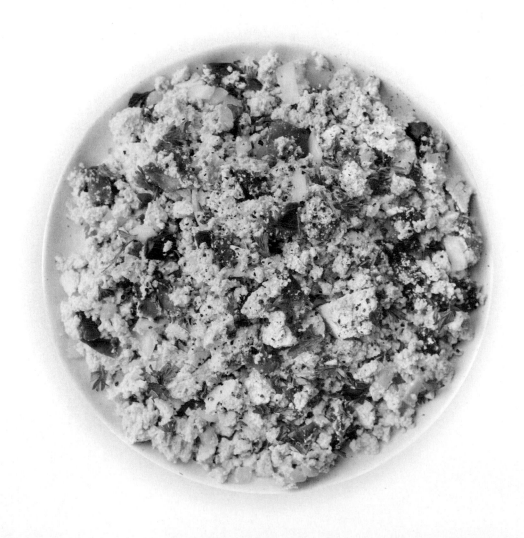

blueberry lemon pancakes

There's no better way to start your weekend than with a stack of fluffy pancakes. Flavored with lemon and sweet in-season blueberries, these pancakes are an all-around delicious and easy breakfast that will quickly become a family favorite.

MAKES 3 servings (about 2 pancakes per serving) ✦ **FROM START TO FINISH:** 20 minutes

1 cup whole wheat flour

1 tablespoon baking powder

Pinch of salt

1 cup unsweetened almond milk

Zest of 1 lemon

1 tablespoon pure maple syrup, plus more for serving

½ cup blueberries, plus more for serving

1. Combine the whole wheat flour, baking powder, and pinch of salt in a bowl. Add the almond milk, lemon zest, and maple syrup and stir until combined. Allow this to sit for 3 minutes and then fold in the blueberries.

2. Heat a nonstick skillet over medium heat, add $1/3$ cup of the batter per pancake, and cook on each side for about 2 minutes, or until browned. Enjoy with maple syrup and more blueberries as desired.

notes

For a gluten-free version, use oat flour.

For a nut-free version, use oat milk or soy milk.

If you do not own a high-quality nonstick pan, you will want to use a small amount of oil to avoid sticking.

**WHOLE WHEAT
FLOUR**

BAKING POWDER

ALMOND MILK

LEMON

MAPLE SYRUP

BLUEBERRIES

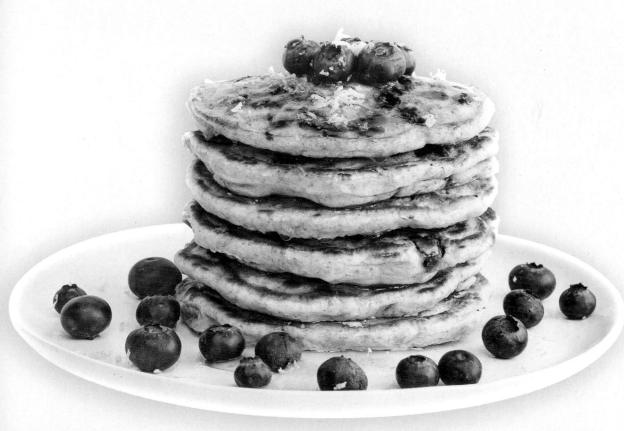

cowboy casanova
breakfast hash

This hash is a versatile recipe that can be equally delicious for breakfast, a pre-prepped lunch, or plant-packed dinner. I love to cook up a batch on a Sunday morning, and send the leftovers with my fiancé to work the next day. Enjoy with Classic Homemade Salsa (page 219), ketchup, Tempeh Bacon (page 52), and the Sunshine Scramble (page 46).

MAKES 4 servings ✦ **FROM START TO FINISH:** 45 minutes

8 Yukon Gold potatoes, unpeeled, chopped

½ medium-size zucchini, chopped

1 red bell pepper, seeded and chopped

½ red onion, diced

½ cup chopped cremini mushrooms

1 (15-ounce) can pinto beans (about 1½ cups), drained and rinsed

1½ teaspoons chili powder

1 teaspoon garlic powder

½ teaspoon sea salt, or to taste

3 garlic cloves, minced

Freshly ground black pepper

1. Preheat the oven to 375°F and line a baking sheet with parchment paper. Spread the potatoes on the baking sheet and bake for 15 minutes.

2. Meanwhile, place the zucchini, bell pepper, onions, mushrooms, beans, chili powder, garlic powder, salt, and garlic in a bowl and toss until the vegetables and beans are coated. Once the potatoes have baked, remove from the oven and add the bean mixture to the pan, spreading out everything evenly with a spatula.

3. Place the pan back in the oven to bake for an additional 15 minutes, or until everything has softened.

4. Pour into a serving dish and add more salt and pepper as desired. Serve with Classic Homemade Salsa (page 219) or ketchup.

YUKON GOLD POTATO

ZUCCHINI

RED BELL PEPPER

RED ONION

CREMINI MUSHROOMS

PINTO BEANS

CHILI POWDER

GARLIC POWDER

GARLIC (CLOVES)

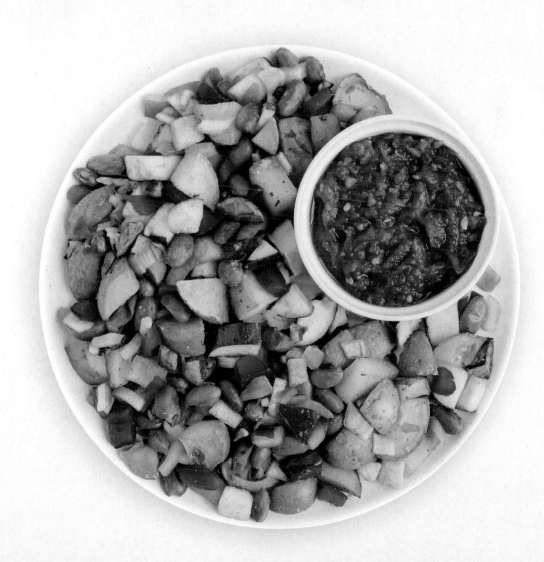

tempeh bacon

Tempeh is a protein-rich food derived from fermented soybeans. While that description may not sound very tasty, tempeh has a nutty, earthy, and meaty flavor you won't be able to get enough of. Similar to its cousin tofu, tempeh takes on flavor very well and can be transformed into a fantastic meat substitute such as this simple bacon, which takes just ten minutes to prepare. Use this as a way healthier substitute for bacon (but just as tasty) in sandwiches, salads, and with your morning breakfast!

MAKES 4 servings (3 slices per serving) ✦ **FROM START TO FINISH:** 10 minutes

2 tablespoons soy sauce

2 tablespoons pure maple syrup

2 teaspoons hot sauce

1 teaspoon ground cumin

1 (8-ounce) package tempeh, sliced into 12 pieces

1. Create a quick marinade by combining the soy sauce, maple syrup, hot sauce, and cumin in a shallow dish. Soak the tempeh in the marinade for about 2 minutes on each side.

2. Place the tempeh in a nonstick pan and cook over medium heat for about 5 minutes on each side, or until crispy.

note If you find tempeh to be too bitter, you can steam it to help offset this. Place the tempeh in a saucepan, cover with water, bring to a boil, lower the heat, and then simmer for 8 to 10 minutes. Cook per the recipe instructions.

SOY SAUCE

MAPLE SYRUP

HOT SAUCE

CUMIN

TEMPEH

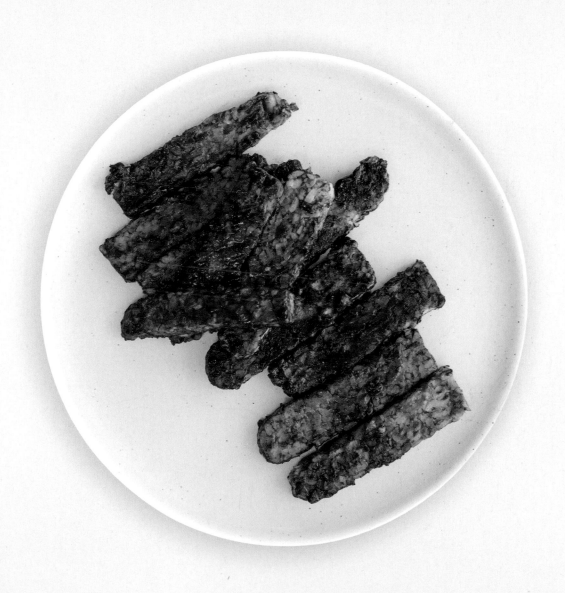

welcome to smoothie land

I like to call smoothies superhero fuel, because they're quick, packed with energy, flooded with nutrients, and most important, one of the most delicious ways to start your day or have an afternoon post-workout pick-me-up. Here are eighteen of my favorite smoothie recipes for every occasion and season.

- **PRO TIP #1:** Drink your smoothie slowly to avoid a blood sugar spike and subsequent crash. Envision eating the contents of your smoothie in a salad bowl for an indication of how long it should take you to drink the full glass.

- **PRO TIP #2:** Always keep frozen sliced and peeled bananas on hand for quick creamy smoothies or nice cream, and to keep your smoothies cold in place of ice.

- **PRO TIP #3:** A high-speed blender, such as a Vitamix, will produce the creamiest, smoothest consistency for your smoothies. With that said, most commercial blenders, from the Ninja to a Bullet, will do the job. You just might want to chop vegetables beforehand and blend for a little longer, to achieve a creamier smoothie.

 In any of these recipes, for a nut-free version, use soy or oat milk, and omit the walnuts.

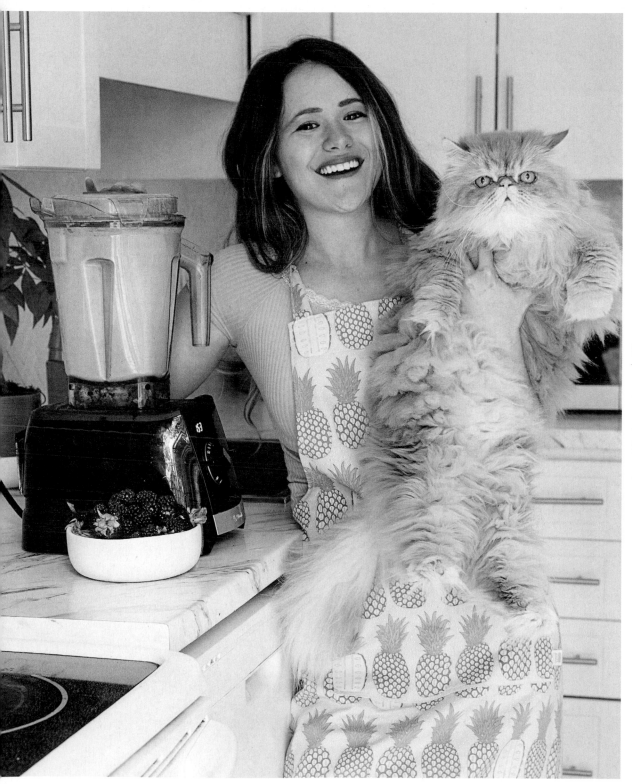

MEAN GREEN SMOOTHIES

I used to be afraid of green smoothies. Yup, even me, a self-proclaimed plant addict, had a hard time finding the courage to try a green-as-the-Hulk blended concoction. I remember suspiciously taking my first sip and being in shock at how good a green smoothie could actually taste! In my Mean Green Smoothies, I've made sure to include a variety of veggies rich in chlorophyll, which is known to help the liver naturally detoxify, provide steady energy, and support your immune system. They're listed from the most "neutral-tasting" to the "meanest and greenest," so you can ease yourself in if you're new to the green smoothie train. Some of these might taste bitter to you at first, but they're worth trying for the amazing nutritional benefits and acquired taste.

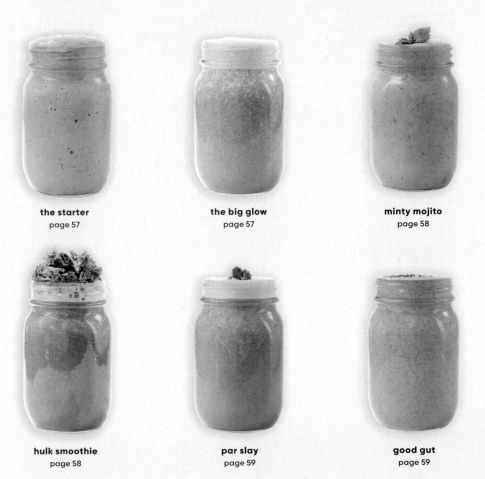

the starter
page 57

the big glow
page 57

minty mojito
page 58

hulk smoothie
page 58

par slay
page 59

good gut
page 59

the starter

MAKES 1 serving ✦ **FROM START TO FINISH:** 5 minutes

1½ cups spinach

1 frozen banana

1 cup unsweetened almond milk

1 tablespoon hemp hearts

Combine all the ingredients in a blender until smooth.

SPINACH   FROZEN BANANA   ALMOND MILK   HEMP HEARTS

the big glow

MAKES 1 serving ✦ **FROM START TO FINISH:** 5 minutes

1 orange, peeled and quartered

1½ cups spinach

1 cup unsweetened almond milk

½ cup frozen pineapple

1 tablespoon chia seeds

Combine all the ingredients in a blender until smooth.

ORANGE   SPINACH   ALMOND MILK   FROZEN PINEAPPLE   CHIA SEEDS

minty mojito

MAKES 1 serving ✦ **FROM START TO FINISH:** 5 minutes

10 fresh mint leaves

2 Medjool dates, soaked for 20 minutes and pitted, or sweetener of choice

Juice of 1 lime

½ medium-size cucumber, peeled

½ cup cold water

¾ cup ice

Combine all the ingredients in a blender until smooth.

MINT   DATES   LIME (JUICE)   CUCUMBER

hulk smoothie

MAKES 1 serving ✦ **FROM START TO FINISH:** 5 minutes

1 cup kale

1 cup frozen chopped mango, peeled

1 cup unsweetened soy milk

1 (½-inch-long) piece fresh ginger, peeled and chopped

Combine all the ingredients in a blender until smooth.

KALE   FROZEN MANGO   SOY MILK   GINGER (FRESH)

par slay

MAKES 1 serving ✦ **FROM START TO FINISH:** 5 minutes

1 cup fresh parsley

1 apple, peeled, cored, and chopped

1 cup unsweetened almond milk

3 Deglet Noor dates, soaked for 20 minutes and pitted, or sweetener of choice

1 teaspoon hemp hearts

Combine all the ingredients in a blender until smooth.

| PARSLEY | APPLE | ALMOND MILK | DATES | HEMP HEARTS |

good gut

MAKES 1 serving ✦ **FROM START TO FINISH:** 5 minutes

1 frozen banana

1 cup spinach

1½ cups unsweetened cashew milk

½ cup broccoli sprouts

¼ avocado, peeled and pitted

1 tablespoon ground flaxseeds

Combine all the ingredients in a blender until smooth.

| FROZEN BANANA | SPINACH | CASHEW MILK | BROCCOLI SPROUTS | AVOCADO | GROUND FLAXSEEDS |

FRUIT-FILLED WONDERS

There are few things more refreshing than a fruity smoothie. I love to maximize the health impact of my fruit smoothies by pairing them with greens, seeds, and spices. All three help regulate a blood sugar spike from the fruit and supercharge your smoothie with more fiber and nutrients. Here are six of my absolute favorites. As you get used to starting your day with a smoothie, I recommend adding a neutral green, such as spinach or chard, to up-level the nutrition value.

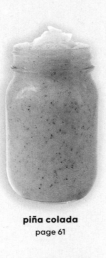

piña colada
page 61

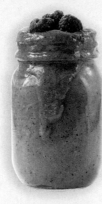

pink elephant
page 61

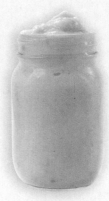

mango tango
page 62

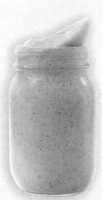

peach cobbler smoothie
page 62

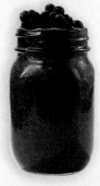

blueberry fields
page 63

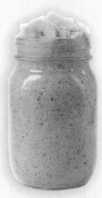

banana mama
page 63

piña colada

MAKES 1 serving ✦ **FROM START TO FINISH:** 5 minutes

1 cup frozen pineapple

¾ cup unsweetened almond milk

¼ cup canned light coconut milk (optional)

¼ teaspoon ground turmeric

1 tablespoon hemp hearts

½ cup ice

Combine all the ingredients in a blender until smooth.

FROZEN PINEAPPLE   ALMOND MILK   COCONUT MILK (OPTIONAL)   TURMERIC   HEMP HEARTS

pink elephant

MAKES 1 serving ✦ **FROM START TO FINISH:** 5 minutes

1½ cups frozen raspberries

1 cup unsweetened almond milk

1 tablespoon chia seeds

1 tablespoon peanut butter

Combine all the ingredients in a blender until smooth.

FROZEN RASPBERRIES   ALMOND MILK   CHIA SEEDS   PEANUT BUTTER

mango tango

MAKES 1 serving ✦ **FROM START TO FINISH:** 5 minutes

2 cups frozen mango

1 cup unsweetened coconut yogurt

½ cup unsweetened almond milk

Combine all the ingredients in a blender until smooth.

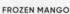

FROZEN MANGO

COCONUT YOGURT

ALMOND MILK

peach cobbler smoothie

MAKES 1 serving ✦ **FROM START TO FINISH:** 5 minutes

2 frozen peaches, pitted but unpeeled
(about 1 cup)

1 cup unsweetened almond milk

¼ cup rolled oats

1 tablespoon hemp hearts

2 Medjool dates, soaked for 20 minutes
and pitted, or sweetener of choice
(optional)

Combine all the ingredients in a blender until smooth.

FROZEN PEACHES

ALMOND MILK

ROLLED OATS

HEMP HEARTS

DATES
(OPTIONAL)

blueberry fields

MAKES 1 serving ✦ FROM START TO FINISH: 5 minutes

1 cup frozen blueberries

1 banana, frozen

1 cup unsweetened almond milk

½ cup unsweetened coconut yogurt

1 tablespoon ground flaxseeds

Combine all the ingredients in a blender until smooth.

FROZEN
BLUEBERRIES

FROZEN BANANA

ALMOND MILK

COCONUT YOGURT

GROUND
FLAXSEEDS

banana mama

MAKES 1 serving ✦ FROM START TO FINISH: 5 minutes

1 frozen banana

1 cup unsweetened almond milk

2 tablespoons shredded unsweetened coconut

2 tablespoons rolled oats

1 tablespoon chia seeds

½ teaspoon pure vanilla extract

Combine all the ingredients in a blender until smooth.

FROZEN
BANANA

ALMOND MILK

COCONUT
FLAKES

ROLLED OATS

CHIA SEEDS

VANILLA
EXTRACT

DECADENT SMOOTHIES

These decadent smoothies are reminiscent of some of my favorite chocolate bars, cakes, and pies, blurring the line between smoothie and dessert. They may taste like heaven, but don't let them fool you! They're also packed with energy, nutrients, and antioxidants to get you through the day. As noted earlier, once you ease yourself into smoothies, it's always great to play around with the nutritional elements, adding neutral greens, such as spinach and chard, where you can!

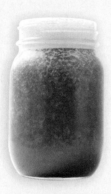

ice capp
page 65

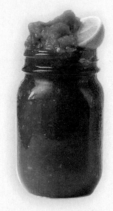

watermelon high slushy
page 65

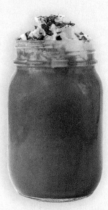

snickers smoothie
page 66

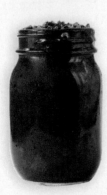

red velvet
page 66

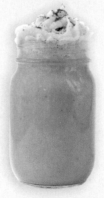

pumpkin pie
page 67

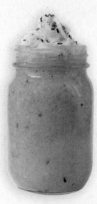

cake batter
page 67

ice capp

MAKES 1 serving ✦ **FROM START TO FINISH:** 5 minutes

1 frozen banana

2 cups ice

1 cup cold brewed coffee

¾ cup unsweetened almond milk

Combine all the ingredients in a blender until smooth.

FROZEN BANANA

BREWED COFFEE

ALMOND MILK

watermelon high slushy

MAKES 1 serving ✦ **FROM START TO FINISH:** 5 minutes

2 cups cubed and seeded watermelon, frozen

Juice of ½ lime

¼ cup ice-cold water

Combine all the ingredients in a blender until smooth.

FROZEN WATERMELON

LIME (JUICE)

snickers smoothie

MAKES 1 serving ✦ **FROM START TO FINISH:** 5 minutes

1 cup unsweetened almond milk

1 frozen banana

1½ tablespoons unsweetened cocoa powder

1½ tablespoons natural peanut butter

1 tablespoon ground flaxseeds

Combine all the ingredients in a blender until smooth.

ALMOND MILK FROZEN BANANA COCOA POWDER PEANUT BUTTER GROUND FLAXSEEDS

red velvet

MAKES 1 serving ✦ **FROM START TO FINISH:** 5 minutes

1 cup frozen pitted cherries

1 cup strawberries, stems removed and frozen

1½ cups unsweetened almond milk

1 tablespoon unsweetened cocoa powder

½ teaspoon pure vanilla extract

Combine all the ingredients in a blender until smooth.

FROZEN CHERRIES FROZEN STRAWBERRIES ALMOND MILK COCOA POWDER VANILLA EXTRACT

pumpkin pie

MAKES 1 serving ✦ FROM START TO FINISH: 5 minutes

1 cup unsweetened oat milk

1 frozen banana

½ cup pure pumpkin puree (not pumpkin pie filling)

1 Medjool date, soaked for 20 minutes and pitted (optional)

1 teaspoon pumpkin pie spice

Combine all the ingredients in a blender until smooth.

OAT MILK   FROZEN BANANA   PUMPKIN PUREE   DATES (OPTIONAL)   PUMPKIN PIE SPICE

cake batter

MAKES 1 serving ✦ FROM START TO FINISH: 5 minutes

1 cup unsweetened cashew milk

1 frozen banana

¼ cup rolled oats

2 regular pitted dates, soaked for 20 minutes (optional)

½ teaspoon pure vanilla extract

1 teaspoon sprinkles (optional)

Combine all the ingredients in a blender until smooth.

CASHEW MILK   FROZEN BANANA   ROLLED OATS   DATES   VANILLA EXTRACT   SPRINKLES (OPTIONAL)

breakfast cookies

Once you start eating cookies for breakfast, it's impossible to go back. Don't worry; just like everything in this cookbook, these cookies are packed with insanely healthy ingredients, such as ground flaxseeds, rolled oats, pumpkin seeds, and more. I've included four varieties to suit every taste. You can store all of these in a sealed container on your counter for up to four days, or freeze for up to one month.

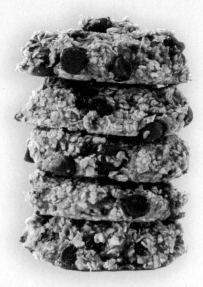

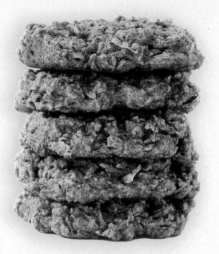

chocolate chip banana bread breakfast cookies
page 70

dreamy zucchini breakfast cookies
page 71

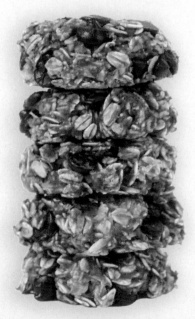

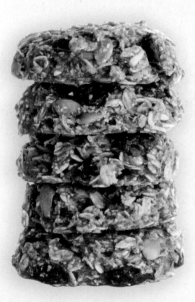

pumpkin breakfast cookies
page 72

nutrient bomb breakfast cookies
page 73

chocolate chip banana bread breakfast cookies

MAKES 8 cookies ✦ **FROM START TO FINISH:** 18 minutes

2 bananas, mashed

1½ cups rolled oats

½ teaspoon ground cinnamon

⅓ cup vegan dark chocolate chips

½ teaspoon baking powder

Pinch of salt

1. Preheat the oven to 375°F and line a baking sheet with parchment paper.

2. Place all the ingredients in a large bowl and mix until fully combined. Wet your hands and form the batter into eight balls. Place at least 1 inch apart on the prepared pan. Flatten the balls with your hands or the back of a fork until they are about ½ inch thick.

3. Bake for 12 minutes, or until a toothpick inserted into a cookie comes out clean.

BANANA

ROLLED OATS

CINNAMON

DARK CHOCOLATE CHIPS

BAKING POWDER

plant-filled mornings

dreamy zucchini breakfast cookies

MAKES 8 cookies ✦ **FROM START TO FINISH:** 18 minutes

¾ cup rolled oats

¼ cup ground flaxseeds

¾ medium-size zucchini, unpeeled, grated, and patted dry (about ¾ cup)

⅓ cup unsweetened almond butter

3 tablespoons pure maple syrup

2 teaspoons ground cinnamon, Ceylon if possible

½ teaspoon baking soda

¼ teaspoon sea salt

½ teaspoon pure vanilla extract

1. Preheat the oven to 375°F and line a baking sheet with parchment paper.

2. Place all the ingredients in a bowl and mix until fully combined. Wet your hands and form the batter into eight balls. Place at least 1 inch apart on the prepared pan. Flatten the balls with your hands or the back of a fork until they are about ½ inch thick.

3. Bake for 12 to 14 minutes, or until a toothpick inserted into a cookie comes out clean.

ROLLED OATS

GROUND FLAXSEEDS

ZUCCHINI

ALMOND BUTTER

MAPLE SYRUP

CINNAMON

BAKING SODA

VANILLA EXTRACT

pumpkin breakfast cookies

MAKES 8 cookies ✦ **FROM START TO FINISH:** 18 minutes

2½ cups rolled oats

1¼ cups pure pumpkin puree (not pumpkin pie filling)

¼ cup pure maple syrup

½ cup vegan dark chocolate chips

½ teaspoon pumpkin pie spice

1 teaspoon pure vanilla extract

1. Preheat the oven to 350°F and line a baking sheet with parchment paper.

2. Place all the ingredients in a bowl and mix until fully combined. Wet your hands and form the batter into eight balls. Place at least 1 inch apart on the prepared pan. Flatten the balls with your hands or the back of a fork until they are about ½ inch thick.

3. Bake for 10 to 12 minutes, or until a toothpick inserted into a cookie comes out clean.

ROLLED OATS

PUMPKIN PUREE

MAPLE SYRUP

DARK CHOCOLATE CHIPS

PUMPKIN PIE SPICE

VANILLA EXTRACT

nutrient bomb breakfast cookies

MAKES 8 cookies ✦ **FROM START TO FINISH:** 20 minutes

1 cup rolled oats

½ cup oat flour

½ cup dried unsweetened cranberries

¼ cup pumpkin seeds

¼ cup ground flaxseeds

1 tablespoon chia seeds

1 teaspoon ground cinnamon, Ceylon if possible

½ teaspoon baking powder

¼ teaspoon salt

2 bananas, mashed

3 tablespoons pure maple syrup

2 tablespoons unsweetened almond milk

1. Preheat the oven to 325°F and line a baking sheet with parchment paper.

2. Mix the oats, oat flour, cranberries, pumpkin seeds, flaxseeds, chia seeds, cinnamon, baking powder, and salt in a large bowl.

3. Stir in the bananas, maple syrup, and almond milk until combined. Set aside for a few minutes, or until the batter has thickened slightly.

4. Wet your hands and form the batter into eight balls. Place at least 1 inch apart on the prepared pan. Flatten the balls with your hands or the back of a fork until they are about ½ inch thick.

5. Bake for 15 to 18 minutes, or until a toothpick inserted into a cookie comes out clean.

ROLLED OATS

OAT FLOUR

DRIED CRANBERRIES

PUMPKIN SEEDS

GROUND FLAXSEEDS

CHIA SEEDS

CINNAMON

BAKING POWDER

BANANA

MAPLE SYRUP

ALMOND MILK

souper bowls

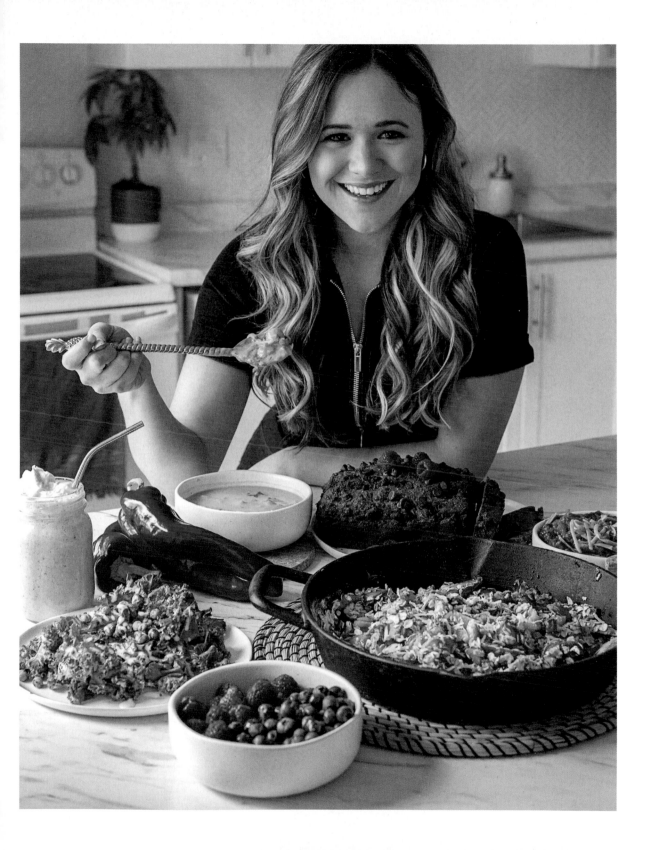

belly-warming minestrone soup

This comforting recipe requires just one pot and a few minutes of prep time to create a nourishing and delicious plant-based soup perfect for lunch or dinner during the workweek. If you are meal prepping this recipe, I always suggest making the pasta separately and heating it up with the soup when you're ready to eat. It keeps it from going soggy in the soup while it's stored in the fridge.

MAKES 4 to 6 servings (2 to 2½ cups per serving) ✦ **FROM START TO FINISH:** 35 minutes

4 garlic cloves, minced

1 medium-size yellow onion, chopped

5 cups vegetable broth

1 (28-ounce) can diced tomatoes (about 3 cups), including liquid

1 (15-ounce) can kidney beans (about 1½ cups), drained and rinsed

1½ cups uncooked whole wheat pasta shells

2 carrots, diced

1 zucchini, diced

¾ cup green beans, chopped

2 teaspoons dried oregano

1 teaspoon freshly squeezed lemon juice

1 cup fresh basil, if available, or spinach

1. Combine the minced garlic and onion with 3 tablespoons of water in a large pot. Sauté over medium heat until the onion is translucent, about 5 minutes.

2. Add all the remaining ingredients, except the fresh basil, to the pot. Bring to a boil, then simmer for 12 to 15 minutes, or until the pasta is cooked. The soup is ready to eat when the pasta is soft and the vegetables are cooked through.

3. Three minutes before the soup is done, add the basil and stir until wilted.

note Make a gluten-free version with brown rice pasta shells.

GARLIC (CLOVES)

YELLOW ONION

VEGETABLE BROTH

DICED TOMATOES

RED KIDNEY BEANS

WHOLE WHEAT SHELLS

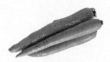
CARROTS

ZUCCHINI

GREEN BEANS

OREGANO

LEMON (JUICE)

BASIL

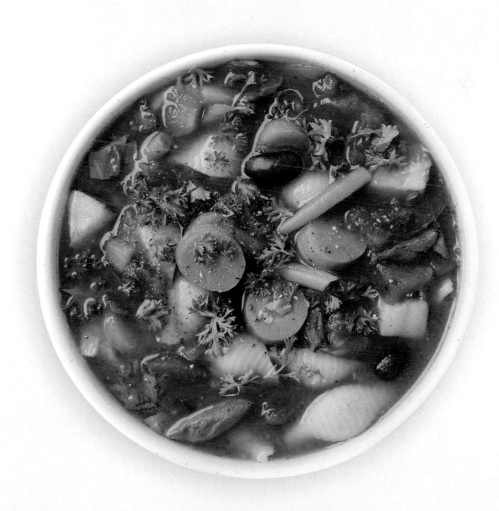

wicked red curry soup

I spent the first twenty years of my life eating the same three cuts of meat in endless rotation. Going plant-based exposed me to such a massive variety of cuisines as well as plants I had never thought of integrating into my diet before. After visiting Thailand in 2017, I fell head over heels in love with Thai red curry. The culture and food in Thailand is heavy on plants and big on flavor. This is my interpretation of a Thai red curry soup, minus the fish sauce and packed with a variety of veggies.

MAKES 4 servings (about 1½ cups per serving) ✦ **FROM START TO FINISH:** 35 minutes

3 garlic cloves, minced

1 medium-size sweet potato, skin on, chopped

1 medium-size yellow onion, diced

½ teaspoon ground ginger

2 tablespoons red curry paste

1 red bell pepper, seeded and chopped

1 cup canned light coconut milk

4 cups vegetable broth

1 teaspoon pure maple syrup

½ cup cremini mushrooms

½ cup frozen green peas

½ cup fresh cilantro, chopped, for serving (optional)

Red onion, finely sliced, for serving (optional)

Juice of ½ lime (optional)

1. Combine the garlic, sweet potato, onion, and ginger with 2 to 3 tablespoons of water in a large pot. Sauté over medium heat for 5 minutes, or until the sweet potatoes have softened slightly.

2. Add the red curry paste and bell pepper to the pot and stir until the paste becomes fragrant, 2 to 3 minutes.

3. Next, add the coconut milk, vegetable broth, maple syrup, and cremini mushrooms. Bring to a boil, then simmer over low heat for 15 to 20 minutes, or until the sweet potatoes are cooked through.

4. Finally, add the green peas and stir until they have thawed. Garnish with the cilantro, red onion, and lime as desired.

GARLIC (CLOVES) **SWEET POTATO** **YELLOW ONION** **GINGER SPICE** **RED CURRY PASTE** **RED BELL PEPPER** **COCONUT MILK**

VEGETABLE BROTH **MAPLE SYRUP** **CREMINI MUSHROOMS** **GREEN PEAS** **CILANTRO (OPTIONAL)** **RED ONION (OPTIONAL)** **LIME JUICE (OPTIONAL)**

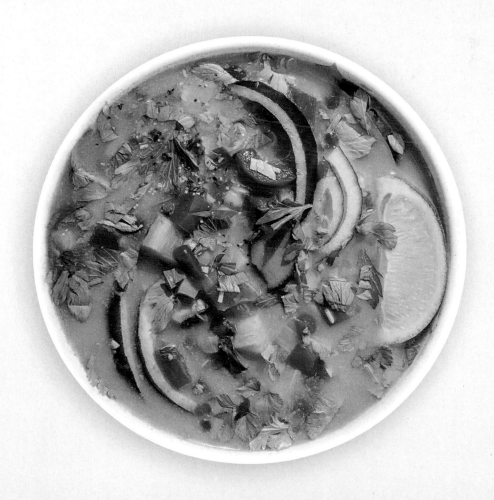

roasted red pepper & cauliflower soup

In vegan recipes, you will often see the creator call for cashews to be soaked overnight. If you don't want to wait twenty-four hours to make a recipe like this amazing soup, I've got a hot tip for you: Simply boil your cashews for fifteen minutes and they'll be nice and soft for pureeing or blending. They make this soup especially creamy.

MAKES 4 servings (about 2 cups per serving) ✦ **FROM START TO FINISH:** 40 minutes

1 medium-size head cauliflower, broken into florets

3 red bell peppers, seeded and sliced

1 yellow onion, sliced

5 garlic cloves, peeled

4 cups vegetable broth

½ cup raw cashews, soaked overnight or boiled for 15 minutes

1 teaspoon smoked paprika

1 teaspoon nutritional yeast

1 teaspoon cider vinegar

1. Preheat the oven to 350°F and line a baking sheet with parchment paper.

2. Place the cauliflower, bell pepper, onion, and garlic on the prepared baking sheet. Bake for 30 minutes, tossing halfway through.

3. Transfer to a large pot along with the remaining ingredients, holding back some of the cauliflower florets to garnish, if desired. Bring to a boil, then simmer, uncovered, for 5 minutes.

4. Allow to cool until safe to handle. Puree with an immersion blender or transfer to a countertop blender and blend until completely smooth.

notes

You can swap out the cashews in this recipe for pine nuts.

For a nut-free version, use white beans, sunflower seeds, or ¼ cup of tahini instead of cashews or pine nuts.

CAULIFLOWER

RED BELL PEPPER

YELLOW ONION

GARLIC (CLOVES)

VEGETABLE BROTH

CASHEWS

SMOKED PAPRIKA

NUTRITIONAL YEAST

CIDER VINEGAR

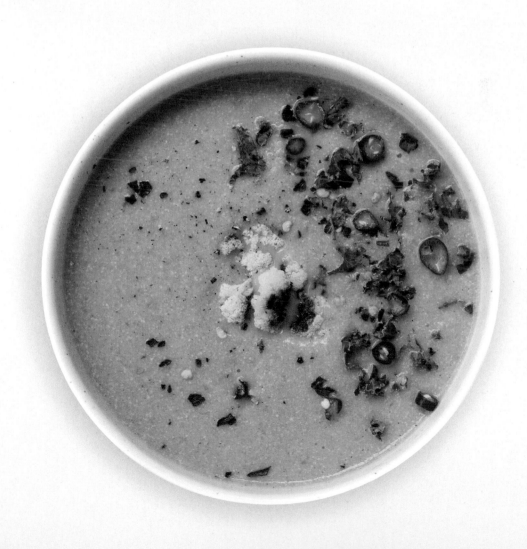

butternut squash soup

For this recipe, I like to buy prefrozen butternut squash chunks. Something about hacking into a big butternut squash just makes my wrist start to ache. If you are buying a butternut squash fresh, you can tell that it's ripe when the skin is hard and it has an even orange color (no green!).

MAKES 4 to 6 servings (about 2½ cups per serving) ✦ **FROM START TO FINISH:** 40 minutes

5 cups chopped frozen or fresh butternut squash (1-inch pieces)

2 carrots, chopped

1 medium-size yellow onion, chopped

4½ cups vegetable broth

2 tablespoons pure maple syrup

3 garlic cloves, peeled

1 teaspoon ground ginger

1 teaspoon salt

½ cup canned light or full-fat coconut milk

1. Combine all the ingredients, except the coconut milk, in a large pot. Bring to a boil, then cover and simmer for 35 minutes, or until the carrots and squash are cooked through.

2. Allow to cool until safe to handle, then puree, using an immersion blender or countertop blender.

3. Stir in the coconut milk, taste, and adjust the seasonings as needed.

BUTTERNUT SQUASH

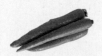

CARROTS

YELLOW ONION

VEGETABLE BROTH

MAPLE SYRUP

GARLIC (CLOVES)

GINGER SPICE

COCONUT MILK

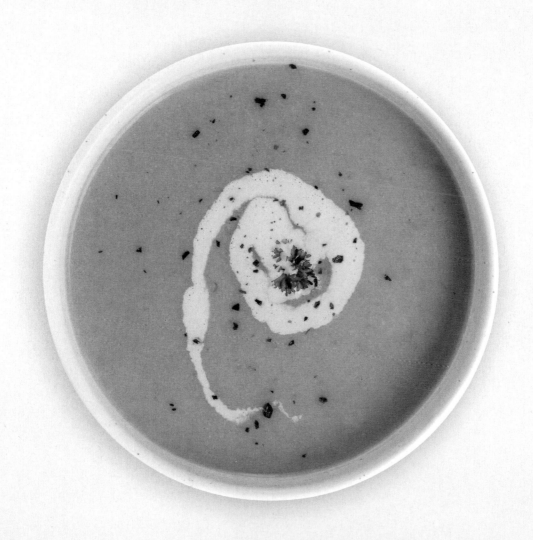

fresh tomato
red lentil bisque

The secret to this bisque is my favorite legume: red lentils. They cook up quickly, are absolutely divine blended into soups and stews, and most important, are packed with fiber, protein, and nutrients. If someone in your family is suspicious of lentils, they are completely undetectable in this bisque, and simply thicken the soup to its signature velvety consistency.

MAKES 4 to 6 servings (about 2 cups per serving) ✦ **FROM START TO FINISH:** 45 minutes

1 medium-size yellow onion, chopped

1 carrot, chopped

3 garlic cloves, peeled and minced

4 cups vegetable broth

10 vine-ripened tomatoes, chopped

1 cup dried red lentils

1 cup fresh basil, if available, or spinach

Salt

1. Combine the onion, carrot, and garlic with 1 to 2 tablespoons of water or vegetable broth, as needed, in a large pot. Sauté over medium heat until the onion becomes translucent, 3 to 5 minutes.

2. Next, add the vegetable broth, tomatoes, and red lentils to the pot. Bring to a boil, then simmer, covered, over low heat for 20 minutes, or until the red lentils are cooked.

3. Allow the soup to cool until it's safe to handle. Add the fresh basil, then puree with an immersion blender or transfer to a high-speed blender to blend until smooth.

4. Taste and adjust the salt as needed.

YELLOW ONION

CARROT

GARLIC (CLOVES)

VEGETABLE BROTH

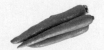

**VINE-RIPENED
TOMATOES**

RED LENTILS

BASIL (FRESH)

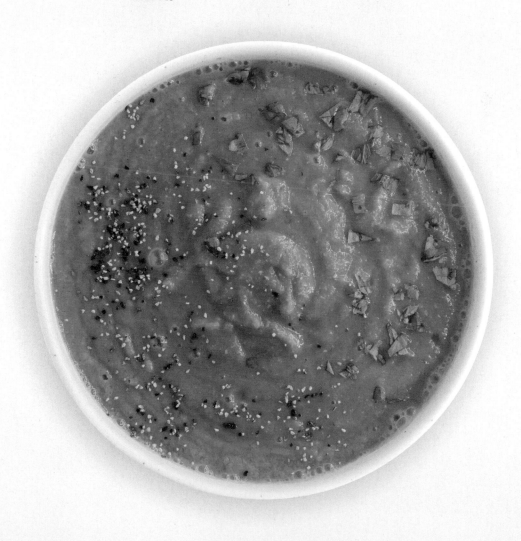

in a jiffy tomato soup

Tomato soup from a can used to be one of my favorite foods while growing up. My dad would add a spoonful of butter to make it especially creamy, and I would top it with lots of pepper and shredded cheese, to boot. This soup is just as quick and creamy as the canned stuff, but way better for you. From start to finish, you can have a big mug of this soup in your hands in less than fifteen minutes.

MAKES 4 servings (about 2 cups per serving) ✦ **FROM START TO FINISH:** 13 minutes

¼ cup raw cashews, soaked overnight or boiled for 15 minutes

2 (28-ounce) cans diced tomatoes (about 6 cups), including liquid

¾ cup unsweetened almond milk

¼ cup fresh basil

1 cup vegetable broth

1 teaspoon onion powder

1 teaspoon garlic powder

1 teaspoon salt

1. Combine all the ingredients in a large pot.

2. Bring to a boil, then simmer, covered, over low heat for 10 minutes.

3. Allow to cool until safe to handle, then use an immersion blender or transfer to a countertop blender and puree until smooth.

note

For a nut-free version, use white beans instead of cashews, and soy milk or rice milk instead of the almond milk.

CASHEWS

DICED TOMATOES

ALMOND MILK

BASIL (FRESH)

VEGETABLE BROTH

ONION POWDER

GARLIC POWDER

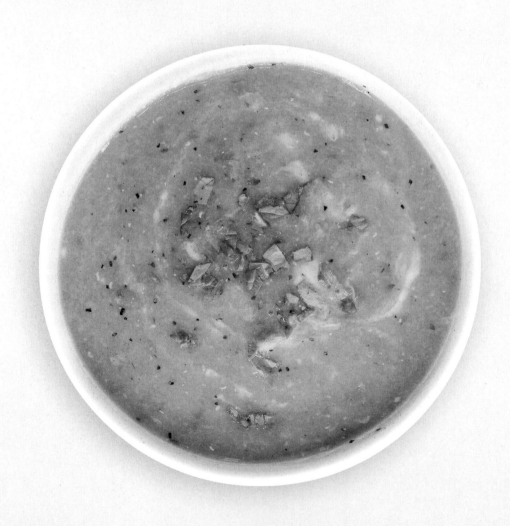

lazy lentil soup

No plant-based cookbook would be complete without a go-to lentil soup. This is the type of recipe to have on hand when you need something especially nourishing, but don't feel like spending hours in the kitchen. Like most of my soup recipes, it comes together with just one pot and accessible ingredients you likely already have in your fridge or pantry.

MAKES 6 to 8 servings (about 2 cups per serving) ✦ **FROM START TO FINISH:** 45 minutes

1 medium-size yellow onion, diced

3 garlic cloves, peeled and minced

2 carrots, diced

2 celery ribs, diced

2 tablespoons balsamic vinegar

1 cup sliced fresh or frozen green beans, cut into 1-inch pieces

4 teaspoons tomato paste

3 medium-size Yukon Gold potatoes, diced

2 cups dried brown or green lentils

1½ teaspoons paprika

½ teaspoon ground cumin

1 teaspoon onion powder

1 tablespoon freshly squeezed lemon juice

8 cups vegetable broth

2 handfuls of spinach

1. Combine the onion and garlic with 2 tablespoons of water in a Dutch oven or large pot. Sauté over medium heat for 3 to 5 minutes, or until the onion starts to become translucent.

2. Next, add the carrots, celery, and balsamic vinegar. Sauté for an additional 3 minutes, stirring to coat the vegetables.

3. Add the green beans, tomato paste, potatoes, lentils, paprika, cumin, onion powder, lemon juice, and vegetable broth. Stir until the soup is well mixed. Bring to a boil, then simmer, covered, over low heat for 30 minutes, stirring occasionally.

4. Finally, add the spinach and stir until it is wilted. Taste and adjust the seasonings as desired.

YELLOW ONION

GARLIC (CLOVES)

CARROTS

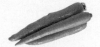

CELERY

BALSAMIC VINEGAR

GREEN BEANS

TOMATO PASTE

YUKON GOLD POTATO

BROWN LENTILS

PAPRIKA

CUMIN

ONION POWDER

LEMON (JUICE)

VEGETABLE BROTH

SPINACH

souper bowls

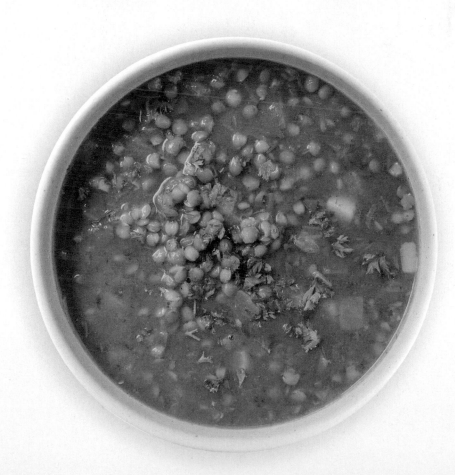

broccoli chedda' soup

After speaking to thousands of vegans over the years, across the board cheese seems to be the most challenging ingredient to part ways with. I don't think there's any plant-based recipe that can completely mimic the taste and texture of cheese, but this soup comes pretty darn close (the secret? Cashews, potato, and paprika!). I love to enjoy this with a big slice of sourdough bread for dipping.

MAKES 4 to 6 servings (about 2 cups per serving) ✦ **FROM START TO FINISH:** 40 minutes

1 red onion, chopped

4 garlic cloves, peeled and minced

1 large carrot, chopped

2 medium-size Yukon Gold potatoes, peeled and chopped

½ cup raw cashews

2 teaspoons paprika

4½ cups vegetable broth

1 large head broccoli, broken into small florets

Salt and freshly ground black pepper (optional)

Red pepper flakes (optional)

1. Combine the onion and garlic with 1 to 2 tablespoons of water in a large pot. Sauté over medium heat until softened, 3 to 5 minutes.

2. Next, add the carrot, potatoes, cashews, paprika, and vegetable broth to the pot. Bring to a boil, then simmer, covered, over low heat for 20 to 25 minutes, or until the potatoes are cooked through.

3. Allow to cool until safe to handle. Use an immersion blender or transfer to a countertop blender and puree until smooth.

4. Pour back into the pot and add the broccoli florets to the soup. Allow to simmer for an additional 8 to 10 minutes, or until the broccoli is cooked through. Taste and add salt, pepper, and red pepper flakes as desired.

RED ONION

GARLIC (CLOVES)

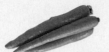

CARROT

YUKON GOLD POTATO

CASHEWS

PAPRIKA

VEGETABLE BROTH

BROCCOLI

RED PEPPER FLAKES
(OPTIONAL)

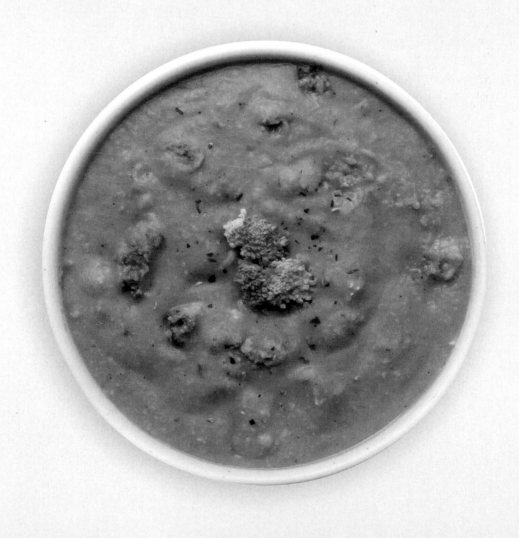

wild rice & lemon soup

With notes of lemon, turmeric, and Italian seasoning, this soup is a delicious dinner or meal prep recipe that will leave your home smelling like a gourmet restaurant. I love this soup because it's extremely versatile as well. If you don't like mushrooms, simply omit or add another veggie, such as zucchini, instead.

MAKES 6 servings (about 1½ cups per serving) ✦ **FROM START TO FINISH:** 45 minutes

6 garlic cloves, peeled and minced

1 medium-size yellow onion, chopped

2 medium-size carrots, peeled and chopped

1 tablespoon lemon zest

¼ teaspoon ground turmeric

1 tablespoon Italian seasoning

5 cups vegetable broth

2 cups chopped cremini mushrooms

¾ cup uncooked wild rice

1½ cups unsweetened almond milk

3 tablespoons freshly squeezed lemon juice

1½ cups kale, chopped

Salt (optional)

1. Combine the garlic and onion with 3 tablespoons of water in a large pot. Sauté over medium heat until the onion starts to become translucent, about 3 minutes.

2. Add the carrots, lemon zest, turmeric, and Italian seasoning to the pot and cook for an additional 3 minutes.

3. Now, add the vegetable broth, mushrooms, and wild rice. Bring to a boil, then simmer, covered, over low heat for 30 minutes, or until the rice has fully cooked.

4. Once the rice is cooked, add the almond milk, lemon juice, and kale. Stir until the kale has wilted. Taste and adjust the salt and seasonings as needed.

 note For a nut-free version, use soy milk instead.

GARLIC (CLOVES)

YELLOW ONION

CARROTS

LEMON (ZEST)

TURMERIC

ITALIAN SEASONING

VEGETABLE BROTH

CREMINI MUSHROOMS

WILD RICE

ALMOND MILK

LEMON (JUICE)

KALE

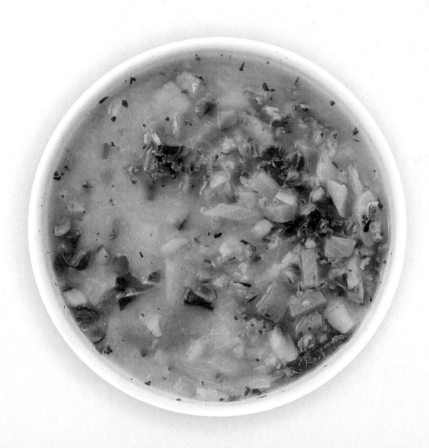

"not your college" ramen

Traditional ramen noodle soup takes two to three days to make with a rich pork and/or beef broth. My college ramen noodle soup was whipped together in a hasty three minutes with a kettle, spice package, and cardboard cup. This ramen is somewhere in between. It's far from authentic, but it does have that delicious umami flavor, thanks to the combination of garlic, ginger, and miso paste. Miso is a fermented food, full of probiotics, which are excellent for gut health. To avoid killing the probiotics with boiling water, you want to add the miso paste after removing your broth from the heat.

MAKES 1 serving ✦ **FROM START TO FINISH:** 15 minutes

BROTH

3 garlic cloves, peeled and minced

1 (½-inch-long) piece fresh ginger, peeled and minced

3 cups water

1 tablespoon cider vinegar

1 tablespoon tahini

1 teaspoon pure maple syrup

1½ cups chopped cremini mushrooms

1 cup spinach

1½ tablespoons brown rice miso paste

1 (85 g) package ramen noodles, spice packet discarded

OPTIONAL TOPPINGS

½ carrot, grated

1 tablespoon sesame seeds

1 chile pepper, chopped

1 green onion, diced

Crushed peanuts

½ cup fresh sprouts

½ cup green peas or edamame

½ cup fresh cilantro

1. Combine the garlic and ginger with 2 tablespoons of water in a large pot. Sauté over medium heat until fragrant, about 2 minutes.

2. Next, add the 3 cups of water along with the cider vinegar, tahini, maple syrup, cremini mushrooms, and spinach to the pot and stir. Simmer for an additional 3 minutes until the mushrooms and spinach have softened.

3. Remove from the heat and whisk in the miso paste until dissolved.

4. To serve, pour the hot broth over the ramen noodles. Cover and allow to sit for at least 3 minutes, or until the noodles have softened. Add your desired vegetable toppings.

GARLIC (CLOVES)

GINGER (FRESH)

CIDER VINEGAR

TAHINI

MAPLE SYRUP

CREMINI MUSHROOMS

SPINACH

MISO PASTE

RAMEN NOODLES

CARROT (OPTIONAL)

SESAME SEEDS (OPTIONAL)

CHILE PEPPER (OPTIONAL)

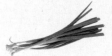
GREEN ONION (OPTIONAL)

PEANUTS (OPTIONAL)

SPROUTS (OPTIONAL)

GREEN PEAS (OPTIONAL)

CILANTRO (OPTIONAL)

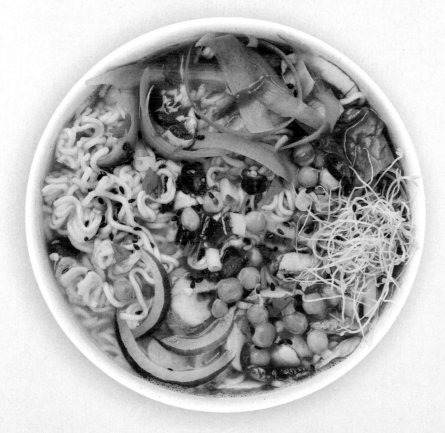

notes

For a gluten-free version, use brown rice vermicelli noodles instead.

For a peanut-free version, omit the crushed peanuts.

chickpea noodle soup

There's some truth to the old wives' tale that a big bowl of soup can help heal a nasty cold. Studies have shown that a hot bowl of soup can relieve nasal congestion while also keeping you hydrated. This soup is always on the menu whenever I feel a cold coming on, and as the meatless version of a chicken noodle soup, it provides such comforting and familiar flavors from my childhood.

MAKES 6 servings (about 2 cups per serving) ✦ **FROM START TO FINISH:** 40 minutes

4 garlic cloves, peeled and minced

1½ medium-size yellow onions, diced

3 celery ribs, diced

2 carrots, peeled and diced

8 cups vegetable broth

3 cups uncooked brown rice fusilli

1 (15-ounce) can chickpeas (about 1½ cups), drained and rinsed

½ teaspoon ground turmeric

1 teaspoon dried thyme

¼ teaspoon sea salt, or more to taste

Freshly ground black pepper

1½ cups spinach

1. Combine the garlic, onions, celery, and carrots with 2 tablespoons of water in a large pot. Sauté over medium heat until softened slightly, about 5 minutes.

2. Add all the remaining ingredients, except the spinach, to the pot, along with black pepper to taste. Bring to a boil, then simmer over low heat for 12 to 15 minutes, or until the pasta is cooked. The soup is ready to eat when the pasta is soft and the vegetables are cooked through.

3. Three minutes before the soup is done, add the spinach and stir until wilted.

note

For meal prep, cook the pasta separately and combine when ready to eat, to prevent it from getting soggy in the fridge.

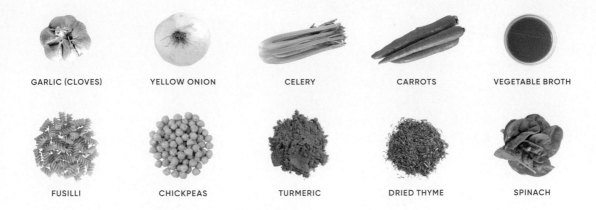

GARLIC (CLOVES) YELLOW ONION CELERY CARROTS VEGETABLE BROTH

FUSILLI CHICKPEAS TURMERIC DRIED THYME SPINACH

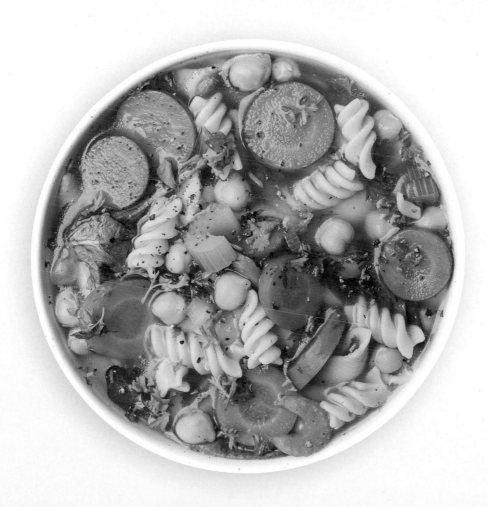

creamy potato leek soup

This is one of the easiest recipes in this cookbook, once you take care of the leeks. Leeks are usually coated in soil when you buy them, with dirt hidden between each layer. Chop them first, discarding the dark green ends and bottom roots, and then place them in a bowl of cold water. Using your hands, work away the dirt in each piece of leek, then scoop out the pieces with a slotted spoon and place in a new, clean bowl. This small step is well worth this delicious warming bowl of soup.

MAKES 4 to 6 servings (about 2 cups per serving) ✦ **FROM START TO FINISH:** 35 minutes

2 leeks, rinsed thoroughly and chopped into 1-inch slices, dark green ends discarded

2 garlic cloves, peeled and minced

4 cups vegetable broth

4 Yukon Gold potatoes, peeled and chopped

1 teaspoon nutritional yeast

½ teaspoon dried thyme

1. Combine the leeks and garlic with a tablespoon of the vegetable broth in a large pot. Sauté over low heat for 8 to 10 minutes, or until softened.

2. Add the chopped potatoes to the pot with the vegetable broth and remaining ingredients. Bring to a boil, then simmer over low heat until the potatoes are soft, about 25 minutes.

3. Remove from the heat and allow to cool until safe to handle. Use an immersion blender or transfer to a countertop blender and puree until smooth.

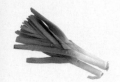

LEEKS

GARLIC (CLOVES)

VEGETABLE
BROTH

YUKON GOLD
POTATO

NUTRITIONAL
YEAST

DRIED THYME

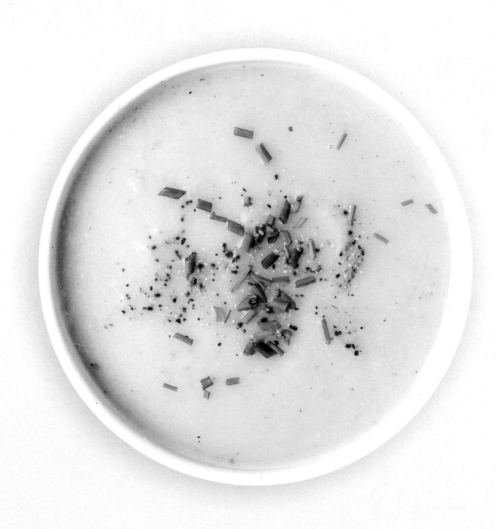

magical mineral broth

Bone broth is one of the latest health fads, touted as a superfood that can help heal digestive issues and drain away inflammation. As plant-based foodies, we know that veggies are far more nourishing than any animal-based broth could ever be. This is why I've created a vegan "bone" broth that is absolutely packed with phytochemicals from rich anti-inflammatory plant-based sources, such as kale, garlic, ginger, turmeric, and beets. Enjoy this for sipping on a cold day, or as a base for cooking up more delicious plant-based dishes.

MAKES 15 to 20 servings ✦ **FROM START TO FINISH:** 2½ hours

8 to 10 quarts filtered water

1 red onion, quartered, with skin

1 sweet potato, cut into chunks

2 cups kale, chopped

4 carrots, chopped

6 garlic cloves, whole

2 bay leaves

2 slices lemon

1 (½-inch-long) piece fresh ginger

1 teaspoon ground turmeric

1 beet, cut into quarters

2 teaspoons sea salt

1. Rinse and scrub the vegetables until clean, leaving the skins on.

2. Place all the ingredients in a large stockpot. Bring to a boil, then simmer, covered, over low heat for up to 2 hours. Taste and adjust the seasonings as needed.

3. Allow to cool until safe to strain. Strain the broth through a mesh sieve into a large enough container, reserving the leftover vegetables for compost, if desired.

4. Allow to cool completely before freezing or storing in the fridge. Will keep in the fridge for up to 5 days, and the freezer for up to 6 months.

note

If you don't have a pot large enough to accommodate 8 quarts of water, you can use the same amount of vegetables, and just half the water.

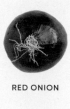

RED ONION

SWEET POTATO

KALE

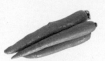

CARROTS

GARLIC (CLOVES)

BAY LEAVES

LEMON (SLICES)

GINGER (FRESH)

TURMERIC

BEET

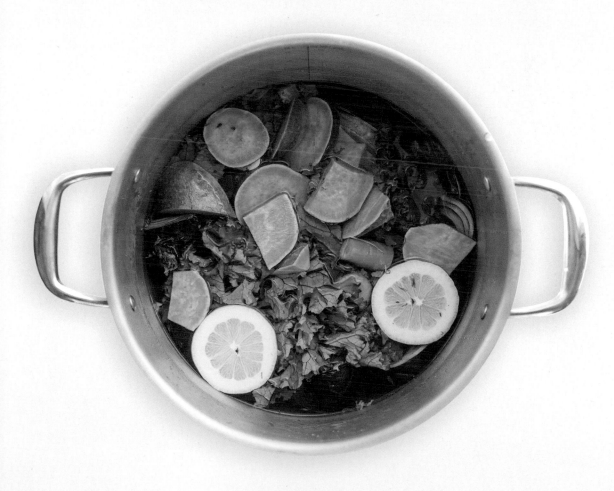

sammys
+ salads

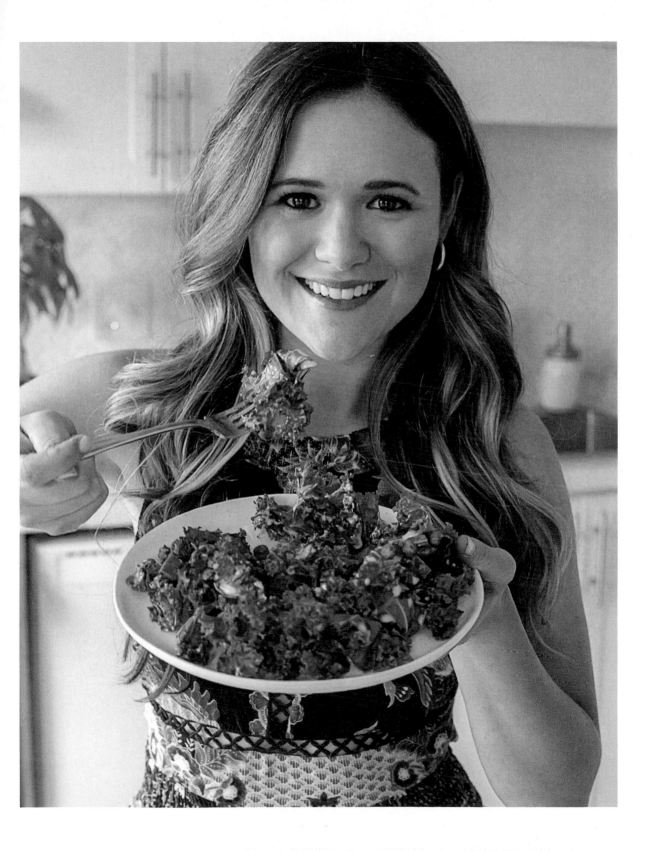

superloaded veggie wrap

This wrap is one of the main reasons I always have hummus and lots of fresh veggies on hand. It's an easy, throw-together lunch or dinner that has the perfect combination of tangy, sweet, savory, and crispy. If you'd rather skip the wrap, this combination makes a killer salad as well.

MAKES 1 serving ✦ **FROM START TO FINISH:** 20 minutes

¼ cup uncooked quinoa

1 cup spinach

1 cup finely chopped iceberg lettuce

½ cup finely chopped red cabbage

¼ cup pickled banana peppers

¼ cucumber, thinly sliced

¼ carrot, peeled and grated

1 handful of broccoli sprouts

1 tablespoon peanuts, crushed

2 tablespoons hummus

1 large whole wheat tortilla wrap

2 tablespoons Go-To Balsamic (page 202)

sammys + salads

1. Cook the quinoa according to the package directions and set aside to cool until room temperature.

2. Place the vegetables, peanuts, and quinoa in a bowl along with the balsamic dressing and toss until well coated.

3. Spread the hummus on the tortilla wrap and pour the quinoa mixture on top. Fold the two ends in, then tightly wrap the tortilla.

notes

For a gluten-free version, make this a salad or use a gluten-free tortilla.

For a peanut-free version, simply omit the crushed peanuts.

QUINOA

SPINACH

LETTUCE

RED CABBAGE

BANANA PEPPERS

CUCUMBER

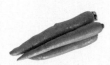

CARROT

BROCCOLI
SPROUTS

PEANUTS

HUMMUS

WHOLE WHEAT
TORTILLA

GO-TO
BALSAMIC

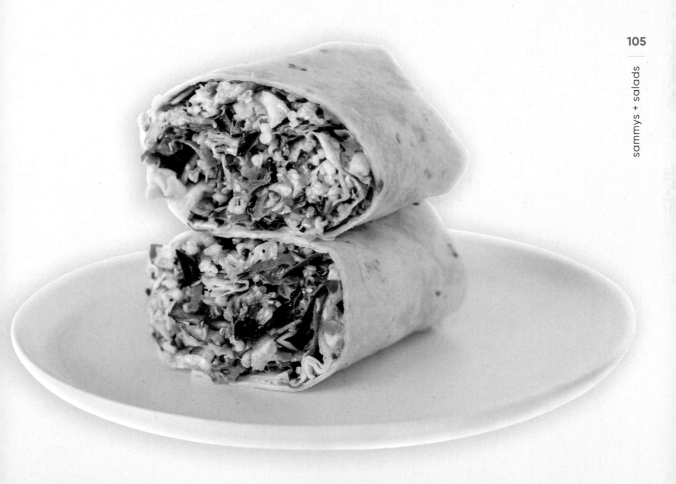

smashed chickpea salad sandwich

The key to this amazing chickpea salad is to "smash" the chickpeas with a potato masher. I first tested it in a food processor, and the consistency was way too mushy. The masher achieves a texture that is similar to a shredded chicken sandwich, plus it's less cleanup too! It's so delicious—you can serve the smashed chickpeas as a salad on its own, as a wrap, or in a sandwich as pictured.

MAKES 2 servings ✦ **FROM START TO FINISH:** 12 minutes

3 tablespoons tahini

2 tablespoons unsweetened soy milk

1 tablespoon pure maple syrup

1 teaspoon cider vinegar

1 teaspoon Dijon mustard

1 teaspoon salt

½ teaspoon dried dill

1 (15-ounce) can chickpeas (about 1½ cups), drained and rinsed

½ red onion, diced

2 green onions, diced

FOR SERVING

4 slices vegan whole wheat sourdough bread

½ cup spinach

½ tomato, sliced

1 handful of broccoli sprouts

1. Whisk together the tahini, soy milk, maple syrup, cider vinegar, Dijon mustard, salt, and dill in a large bowl until smooth.

2. Add the chickpeas, red onion, and green onions to the bowl, and crush with a potato masher until you get a thick, moldable consistency.

3. Stir until the tahini sauce and crushed chickpeas are combined. Taste and adjust the seasonings as needed.

4. Serve on sourdough bread with your toppings of choice.

note Make a gluten-free version with your favorite gluten-free bread.

TAHINI

SOY MILK

MAPLE SYRUP

CIDER VINEGAR

DIJON MUSTARD

DRIED DILL

CHICKPEAS

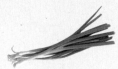

RED ONION

GREEN ONION

SOURDOUGH BREAD

SPINACH

TOMATO

BROCCOLI SPROUTS

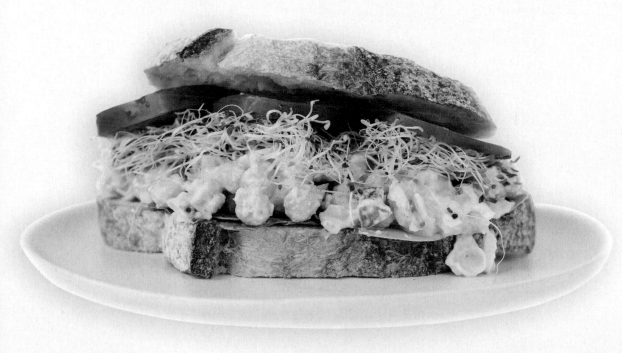

tlt (tempeh, lettuce, tomato)

Toasted sourdough bread, crisp lettuce, marinated tempeh bacon, sweet sliced tomato, and a tangy cashew mayo—you're sure to fall head over heels in love with this TLT. Best enjoyed in the summer with a cold beverage in hand and your feet up after a long day.

MAKES 1 serving ✦ **FROM START TO FINISH:** 20 minutes

2 slices vegan sourdough bread

1 serving Cashew Mayo (page 207)

½ cup shredded lettuce

½ tomato, sliced

6 slices Tempeh Bacon (page 52)

To assemble the sandwich, spread the cashew mayo on both slices of bread. Then layer with the lettuce, tomato, and tempeh bacon.

note

To make a gluten-free version, use gluten-free bread instead, or layer the ingredients on a base of arugula.

SOURDOUGH BREAD

CASHEW MAYO

LETTUCE

TOMATO

TEMPEH BACON

sammys + salads

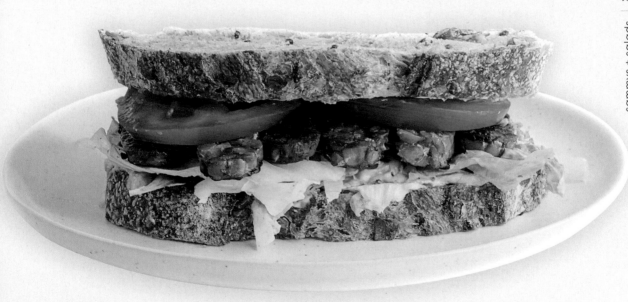

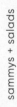

buffalo chick'n wrap

My love for buffalo hot sauce runs deep. I could add it to just about any savory dish, but it's particularly amazing in this wrap. For chicken, we trade in a simple battered tofu that could also be used for nuggets or fingers, if desired.

MAKES 2 servings ✦ **FROM START TO FINISH:** 35 minutes

½ cup unsweetened almond milk

½ cup vegan panko bread crumbs

8 ounces extra-firm tofu, pressed

6 tablespoons hot sauce

¼ cup hummus or other dressing of choice

2 whole wheat tortillas

1 cup shredded iceberg lettuce

1 red onion, diced

1 carrot, grated

½ cup broccoli sprouts

1. Preheat the oven to 350°F and line a baking sheet with parchment paper.

2. Place the almond milk and bread crumbs into two separate shallow bowls. Slice the pressed tofu into 1-inch-wide strips, dip into the almond milk, then coat with the bread crumbs. Place in a single layer on the baking sheet.

3. Bake for 10 minutes, then flip the tofu and bake for an additional 10 minutes, or until crispy.

4. Place the buffalo tofu strips in a bowl and toss with the hot sauce until coated.

5. Spread the hummus or dressing of choice on each tortilla, and add the iceberg lettuce, red onion, carrot, broccoli sprouts, and buffalo tofu strips. Fold in the sides of the tortilla, and tightly roll.

notes

These chick'n strips are wonderful on their own as well, or as leftovers. Make more for later by using the entire package of tofu, and doubling the panko and almond milk batter.

Make a gluten-free version by using gluten-free panko and serving on top of a bed of greens.

For a nut-free version, use soy or rice milk instead of almond milk.

ALMOND MILK

PANKO BREAD
CRUMBS

EXTRA-FIRM TOFU

HOT SAUCE

HUMMUS

WHOLE WHEAT
TORTILLA

LETTUCE

RED ONION

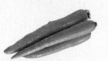

CARROT

BROCCOLI SPROUTS

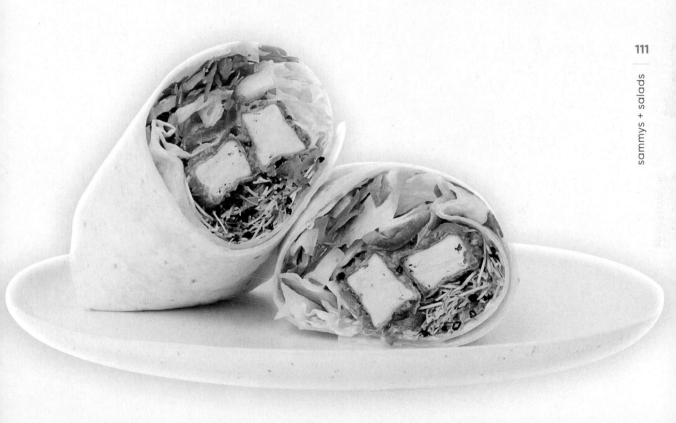

garden of life pita pizza

Everyone needs a five-minute lunch in their plant-based meal arsenal, and this pita pizza perfectly fits the bill. This recipe is a mouthwatering combo of luscious beet hummus, arugula, pickled onions, and cherry tomatoes all piled high on a whole-grain pita. I top this with pine nuts, but you can swap in walnuts, if you prefer.

MAKES 1 serving ✦ **FROM START TO FINISH:** 5 minutes

3 tablespoons Beet Hummus (page 198)

1 whole wheat pita

1 cup arugula

¼ cup Quick Pickled Red Onions (page 226)

4 cherry tomatoes

3 tablespoons pine nuts or walnuts

Spread a thick layer of beet hummus onto the whole wheat pita, and top with the arugula, pickled onions, cherry tomatoes, and pine nuts. Enjoy immediately.

notes

For a gluten-free version, use a gluten-free pita or gluten-free vegan flatbread instead.

For a nut-free version, simply omit the pine nuts.

BEET HUMMUS

PITA BREAD

ARUGULA

**QUICK PICKLED
RED ONIONS**

**CHERRY
TOMATOES**

PINE NUTS

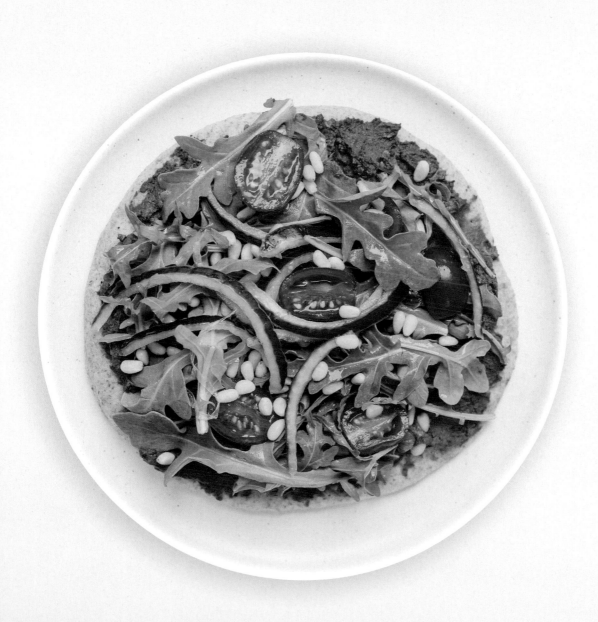

build-a-bowl

For this recipe, I use a basic formula of greens, proteins, carbs, veggies, crunch, and sauce with hopes of inspiring you to create your own nourishing bowl full of ingredients you love. Using these basic building blocks, the combinations are literally endless for the amazing bowls you can make using just whole food, plant-based ingredients. I've included some of my favorites here.

MAKES 1 serving ✦ **FROM START TO FINISH:** 30 minutes

¼ cup uncooked quinoa

1½ cups arugula

½ cup canned chickpeas, drained and rinsed

½ avocado, peeled, pitted, and sliced

½ red bell pepper, seeded and thinly sliced

½ carrot, ribboned

½ jalapeño pepper, sliced

1 tablespoon hemp hearts

1 serving Turmeric Tahini Dressing (page 204)

1. Cook the quinoa according to the package directions, and allow it to cool to room temperature.

2. Combine all the ingredients, except the dressing, in a bowl, and when ready to serve, drizzle the Turmeric Tahini Dressing over the top.

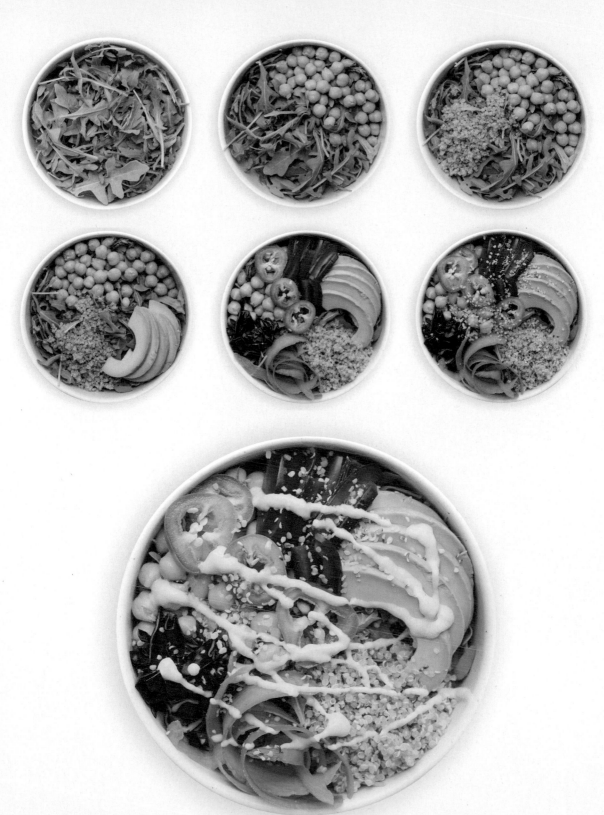

beaming burrito bowl

Burrito bowls are one of the best plant-based recipes to meal prep because they're insanely easy and customizable. You can swap out just about any of the listed ingredients for ones you fancy more, and it will still be delicious, filling, and nourishing. Pinto beans instead of black beans? Sure! Quinoa instead of wild rice? Why not! Eggplant instead of sweet potato? Go for it! I think you catch the drift.

MAKES 4 servings ✦ **FROM START TO FINISH:** 45 minutes

1 large sweet potato, unpeeled, chopped

1 medium-size yellow onion, chopped

1 red bell pepper, seeded and chopped

1 teaspoon ground cumin

1 teaspoon chili powder

Salt

1 cup uncooked wild rice

1 (15-ounce) can black beans (about 1½ cups), drained and rinsed

4 servings Vegan Queso (page 214)

1 avocado, peeled, pitted, and sliced

3 tablespoons pumpkin seeds

¼ cup fresh cilantro, chopped

1. Preheat the oven to 400°F and line a baking sheet with parchment paper. Place the sweet potato, onion, and bell pepper on the prepared baking sheet, and season with the cumin, chili powder, and salt to taste, ensuring the vegetables are covered evenly. Bake for about 35 minutes, or until the sweet potato is cooked through.

2. Meanwhile, cook the wild rice according to the package directions.

3. Divide the rice equally among the bowls, and top with the sweet potato mixture, beans, Vegan Queso, sliced avocado, pumpkin seeds, and cilantro for garnish.

SWEET POTATO

YELLOW ONION

RED BELL PEPPER

CUMIN

CHILI POWDER

WILD RICE

BLACK BEANS

VEGAN QUESO

AVOCADO

PUMPKIN SEEDS

CILANTRO

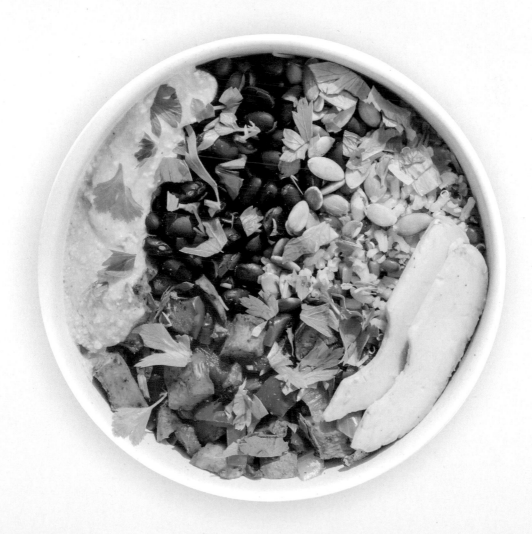

tangy potato salad

You will never believe that the base of the sauce in this potato salad is made from white beans! Not only are white beans a legume packed with fiber and protein, they can also be blended into a velvety sauce mimicking mayo or cream. Pair it with cider vinegar, garlic, and sea salt and you've got a winning combo for a delicious picnic-perfect potato salad.

MAKES 6 servings ✦ **FROM START TO FINISH:** 35 minutes

2 pounds mini red potatoes, quartered

Salt and freshly ground black pepper

1 (15-ounce) can white, navy, or kidney beans (about 1½ cups), drained and rinsed

1 teaspoon Dijon mustard

1½ teaspoons cider vinegar

1 teaspoon sea salt

½ teaspoon garlic powder

½ cup chopped dill pickle

1 red bell pepper, seeded and diced

2 tablespoons chopped fresh dill

½ red onion, chopped

1. Preheat the oven to 400°F and line a baking sheet with parchment paper.

2. Spread the quartered red potatoes on the prepared baking sheet with a pinch of salt and pepper, and roast for about 25 minutes, or until slightly crispy.

3. While the potatoes are roasting, make the dressing: In a countertop blender, combine the beans, Dijon mustard, cider vinegar, sea salt, and garlic powder. Blend until combined, then taste and adjust the seasonings as needed.

4. Allow the potatoes to cool, then combine them in a bowl with the dressing and the remaining ingredients. Enjoy immediately or cover and refrigerate for up to 3 days.

MINI RED POTATOES

WHITE BEANS

DIJON MUSTARD

CIDER VINEGAR

GARLIC POWDER

PICKLE

RED BELL PEPPER

FRESH DILL

RED ONION

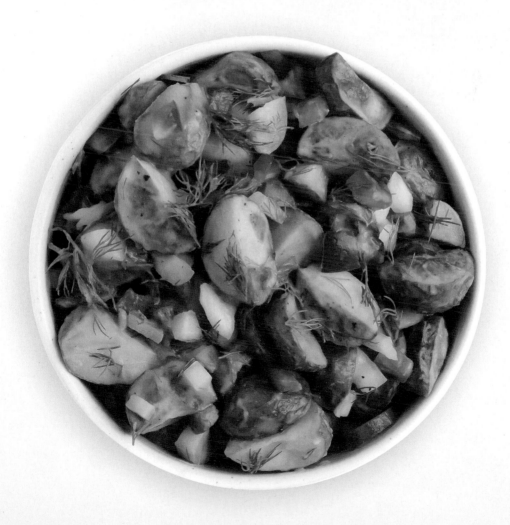

balsamic pasta salad

This simple pasta salad is the perfect barbecue or picnic dish that's sure to impress a crowd. The blend of citrusy cherry tomatoes, artichoke hearts, and fresh, sweet basil creates an amazing combination for spring or summer. Just make sure to add the salad dressing when you're ready to eat.

MAKES 6 servings ✦ **FROM START TO FINISH:** 25 minutes

1 (12-ounce) package whole-grain rotini pasta

2½ cups cherry tomatoes, sliced in half

¼ cup water

1 cup fresh basil, chopped

2 cups spinach, chopped

1 cup artichoke hearts (canned or jarred in brine or water), chopped

1 cup pitted Kalamata olives

6 tablespoons Go-To Balsamic (page 202)

1. Cook the pasta according to the package directions. Drain and rinse in cold water until cooled to room temperature.

2. Meanwhile, combine the cherry tomatoes with ¼ cup of water in a skillet. Cover and let cook over medium heat until the tomatoes begin to burst, about 6 minutes.

3. Combine the cooled pasta with all the vegetables in a bowl, add the balsamic dressing, and toss lightly until coated. Enjoy immediately.

4. If serving later, store the pasta mixture in the fridge separate from the dressing for up to 3 days. When ready to serve, pour the balsamic dressing over the top and toss.

note

For a gluten-free version, use brown rice or chickpea pasta instead.

ROTINI

CHERRY TOMATOES

BASIL (FRESH)

SPINACH

ARTICHOKES

OLIVES (KALAMATA)

GO-TO BALSAMIC

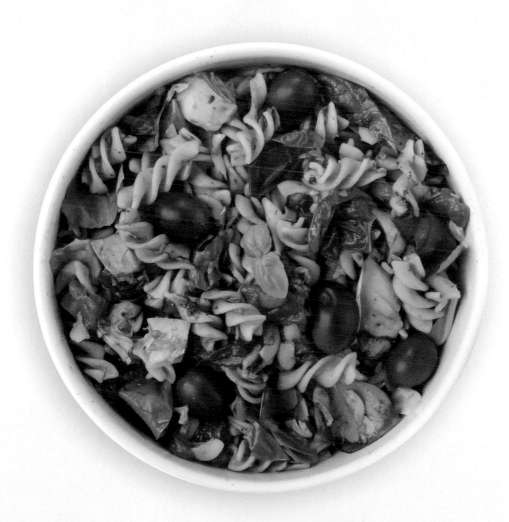

sammys + salads

crunchy peanut shredded salad

I have to admit, I was never a huge fan of salads until just a few years ago. They never felt satisfying enough to take for lunch or eat as a quick dinner, and I was always left wanting something more. If you're anything like I was, I'm confident this salad will flip the switch for you. It's savory, sweet, crunchy, and tangy all in one, with an amazing creamy peanut dressing.

MAKES 4 servings ✦ **FROM START TO FINISH:** 25 minutes

1 cup uncooked quinoa

2 cups finely shredded purple cabbage

1 large carrot, peeled and grated

1 red bell pepper, seeded and thinly sliced

½ large cucumber, seeded and thinly sliced

1 cup fresh cilantro, chopped

3 green onions, chopped

¼ cup crushed peanuts

4 servings Spicy Peanut Dressing (page 203)

1. Cook the quinoa according to the package directions. Set aside and allow to cool.

2. Combine the quinoa with all the remaining ingredients, except the dressing, in a large serving bowl and toss. Drizzle the peanut dressing over the top when ready to serve.

note

For a peanut-free version, use hemp seeds in place of the peanuts and Go-To Balsamic (page 202) instead of the peanut dressing.

QUINOA

PURPLE CABBAGE

CARROT

RED BELL PEPPER

CUCUMBER

CILANTRO

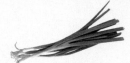

GREEN ONIONS

PEANUTS

SPICY PEANUT DRESSING

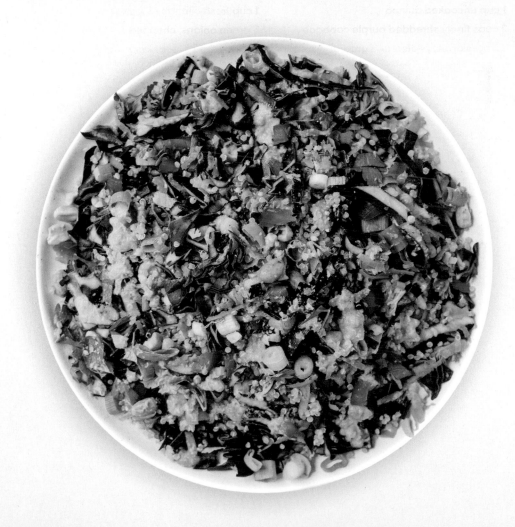

cool ranch kale salad

The key to an amazing kale salad is giving it a deep tissue massage. I'm not kidding! Gently massaging the kale with your hands and a bit of lemon juice helps break down the cell structure of kale, resulting in a softer texture and less bitter flavor. It's even better when it's smothered in my Creamy Ranch Dressing (page 206) and topped with crispy chickpeas.

MAKES 4 servings ✦ **FROM START TO FINISH:** 35 minutes

1 (15-ounce) can chickpeas (about 1½ cups), drained and rinsed

½ teaspoon garlic powder

½ teaspoon paprika

½ teaspoon cider vinegar

½ teaspoon salt

6 cups curly kale, chopped

1 tablespoon freshly squeezed lemon juice

4 servings Creamy Ranch Dressing (page 206)

1 tablespoon hemp hearts (optional)

1. Preheat the oven to 375°F and line a baking sheet with parchment paper.

2. Toss the chickpeas with the garlic powder, paprika, cider vinegar, and salt in a large bowl, until coated. Pour the seasoned chickpeas onto the prepared baking sheet and bake for about 25 minutes, until crispy.

3. Combine the kale and lemon juice in a large serving bowl and massage until softened slightly, 2 to 3 minutes. Add the ranch dressing and toss, then pour the crispy chickpeas over the top. Garnish with hemp hearts, as desired.

CHICKPEAS

GARLIC POWDER

PAPRIKA

CIDER VINEGAR

KALE

LEMON (JUICE)

CREAMY RANCH
DRESSING

HEMP HEARTS
(OPTIONAL)

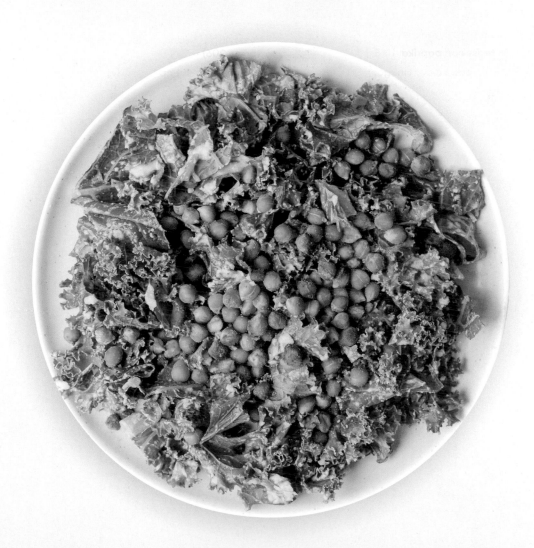

citrus solstice salad

Want to supercharge your salad with nutrients? Add broccoli sprouts! Just one serving contains a hundred times higher concentration of sulforaphane, a powerful compound found in cruciferous vegetables, than does broccoli itself. It's widely touted as anticarcinogenic and anti-inflammatory, and is thought to support heart and brain health. This simple salad plays on the bitterness of the arugula, broccoli sprouts, and radishes, offset with the sweet note of clementine and a balsamic drizzle.

MAKES 1 serving ✦ **FROM START TO FINISH:** 10 minutes

3 cups arugula

1 clementine, peeled and separated

2 radishes, sliced

1 handful of broccoli sprouts

2 tablespoons crushed walnuts

2 tablespoons balsamic glaze or reduction

1. Toss together the arugula, clementine, radishes, and broccoli sprouts in a large serving bowl.

2. Sprinkle with the crushed walnuts, and finish with a balsamic glaze when ready to serve.

notes

Make a nut-free version by using pumpkin seeds instead of walnuts, or simply omitting.

Balsamic glaze or reduction is available at most grocery stores.

ARUGULA   CLEMENTINE   RADISHES   BROCCOLI   WALNUTS   BALSAMIC GLAZE
                                                       SPROUTS

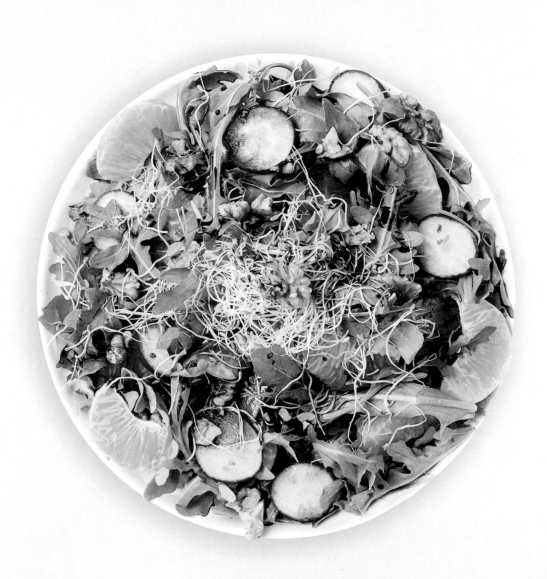

quinoa cranberry
harvest salad

Reminiscent of the changing colors of fall, this salad is the perfect accompaniment to Thanksgiving dinner. Packed with fiber and protein-rich quinoa, sweet potato, dried cranberries, and my tangy Apple Cider Vinaigrette (page 202), it also makes a wonderful lunch for the workweek.

MAKES 4 servings ✦ **FROM START TO FINISH:** 35 minutes

1½ medium-size to large sweet potatoes, unpeeled, diced

¾ cup uncooked quinoa

2 cups kale, massaged for 2 to 3 minutes, or until tender (see salad directions on page 124 for how to massage)

½ cup dried cranberries

¼ cup pumpkin seeds

4 servings Apple Cider Vinaigrette (page 202)

1. Preheat the oven to 400°F and line a baking sheet with parchment paper.

2. Place the sweet potatoes on the prepared baking sheet and roast for 25 minutes until soft.

3. Meanwhile, cook the quinoa according to the package directions.

4. Allow the sweet potato and quinoa to cool to room temperature before combining all the ingredients, except the dressing, in a large bowl. Refrigerate until ready to serve, and drizzle with the cider vinegar dressing.

SWEET POTATO

QUINOA

KALE

**DRIED
CRANBERRIES**

PUMPKIN SEEDS

**APPLE CIDER
VINAIGRETTE**

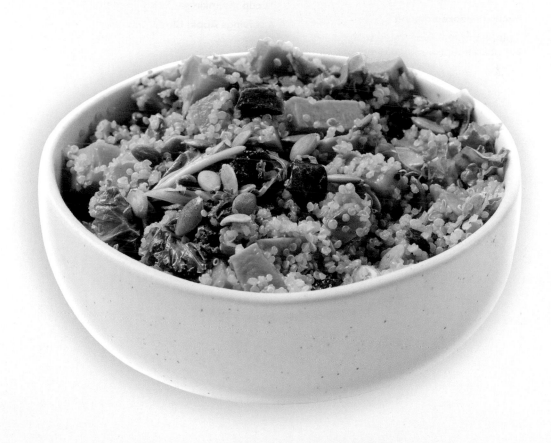

roasted corn, bell pepper & cilantro salad

Every summer, I love to pick up sweet corn on the cob from our local farm stand. It's only around for a few short weeks, and this salad is on quick rotation as we savor those fresh seasonal flavors. If corn is out of season, you can substitute frozen corn kernels.

MAKES 4 servings ✦ **FROM START TO FINISH:** 15 minutes

4 ears of corn, husked with silks removed, or 2½ cups frozen corn kernels

⅓ cup vegetable broth

2 red bell peppers, seeded and chopped

1 red onion, chopped

2 cups fresh cilantro, chopped

1 avocado, peeled, pitted, and diced

4 servings Cilantro Lime Dressing (page 205)

1. Carefully cut the kernels off the ears of corn. Combine the corn kernels with the vegetable broth in a skillet and sauté for 3 to 5 minutes.

2. Toss together the bell peppers, red onion, cilantro, avocado, and cooked corn. When ready to eat, drizzle with the Cilantro Lime Dressing.

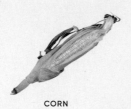

CORN

VEGETABLE BROTH

RED BELL PEPPER

RED ONION

CILANTRO

AVOCADO

CILANTRO LIME
DRESSING

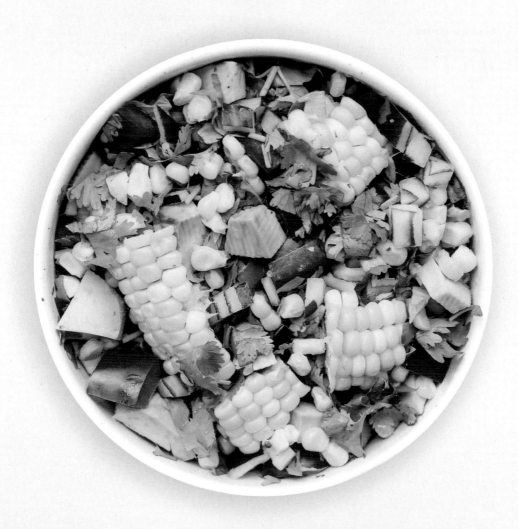

CHAPTER

4

the main event

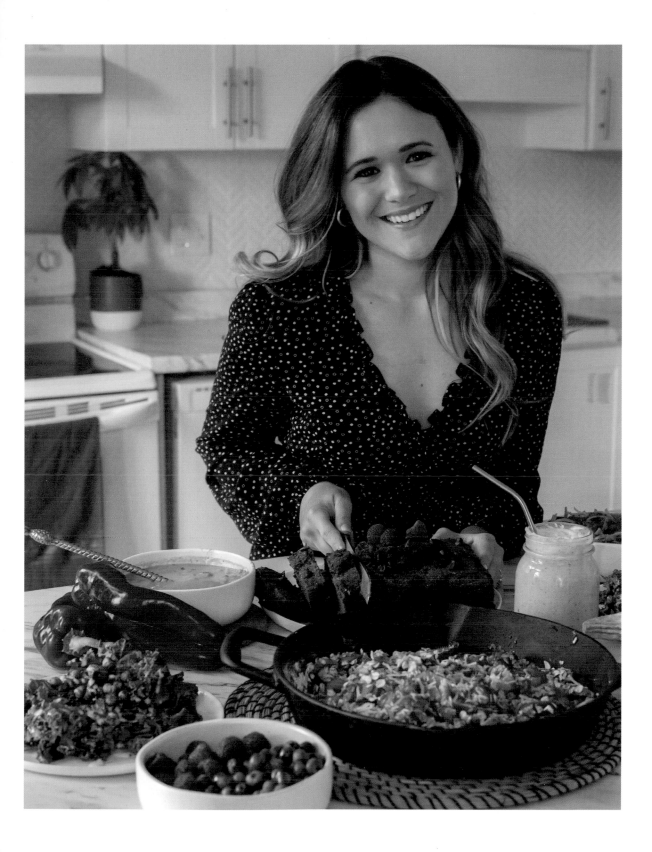

presto pesto penne

Basil is quite possibly my favorite herb. It has such a recognizable, sweet flavor, and when paired with pine nuts, tomato, garlic, lemon juice, and a bit of sea salt, it's brought to a whole other level of deliciousness. If you can't source pine nuts at your local grocery store, feel free to replace them with cashews in this recipe. I've even made it with white beans in a pinch (just use ¾ cup of the beans instead of the pine nuts)!

MAKES 4 servings ✦ **FROM START TO FINISH:** 25 minutes

1 (16-ounce) package whole wheat penne (about 2 cups)

2 cups fresh sweet basil

2 cups spinach

3 garlic cloves, peeled

1 vine-ripened tomato

2 tablespoons freshly squeezed lemon juice

1 teaspoon salt

¾ cup raw pine nuts

1 cup cherry tomatoes, sliced in half

1. Cook the pasta according to the package directions; keep warm.

2. **Meanwhile, make the pesto:** Combine the basil, spinach, garlic, tomato, lemon juice, and salt in a food processor and process until smooth.

3. Add the pine nuts and process again until a smooth pesto is formed. Taste and adjust the salt level as desired.

4. In a large bowl, mix the warm pasta with the pesto and halved cherry tomatoes.

notes

For a gluten-free version, use brown rice penne or rotini instead.

For a nut-free version, swap out the pine nuts for white beans instead.

PENNE

BASIL (FRESH)

SPINACH

GARLIC (CLOVES)

VINE-RIPENED TOMATOES

LEMON (JUICE)

PINE NUTS

CHERRY TOMATOES

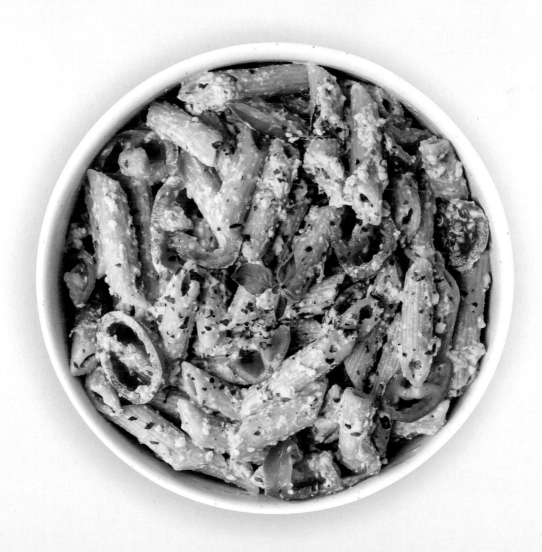

garlic lovers' vegan alfredo

If any recipe in this cookbook is a labor of love, this vegan Alfredo would be considered it. This recipe requires a few moving parts, but is well worth the beautiful explosion of flavor when it all comes together. And good news: roasting garlic actually reduces the pungent smell (and subsequent garlic breath) that often accompanies garlic-heavy dishes.

MAKES 4 servings ✦ **FROM START TO FINISH:** 50 minutes

4 whole heads garlic

1 head broccoli, chopped into florets

1 cup cremini mushrooms

¼ cup vegetable broth

1 (16-ounce) package whole-grain fettuccine

¼ cup unsweetened soy milk

1 teaspoon cider vinegar

½ teaspoon salt, plus more to serve

Fresh parsley, to serve

Red pepper flakes, to serve

Freshly ground black pepper, to serve

1. Preheat the oven to 400°F.

2. Using a sharp knife, slice ½ inch off the top of the whole heads of garlic, exposing the surface of the individual cloves. Wrap the whole heads in foil, place in the middle rack of the oven, and bake for 35 to 40 minutes, or until softened.

3. Combine the broccoli and mushrooms with the vegetable broth in a large skillet and sauté over medium heat until softened, about 6 minutes.

4. Cook the pasta according to the package directions. Before draining, save ½ cup of the pasta water.

5. Meanwhile, remove the garlic heads from the oven and unwrap the foil. Allow to cool enough to be handled before squeezing the heads into a bowl, discarding the skins once finished. Add the soy milk, cider vinegar, and salt to the garlic and whisk until a creamy sauce is formed.

6. Add the garlic sauce to the broccoli mixture, along with the reserved pasta water, and stir until well incorporated. Slowly add the cooked fettuccine and stir until coated.

7. Enjoy immediately with fresh parsley, red pepper flakes, and salt and black pepper to taste.

note For a gluten-free version, use brown rice fettuccine.

GARLIC (HEAD)

BROCCOLI

CREMINI MUSHROOMS

VEGETABLE BROTH

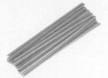

FETTUCCINE

SOY MILK

CIDER VINEGAR

FRESH PARSLEY

RED PEPPER FLAKES

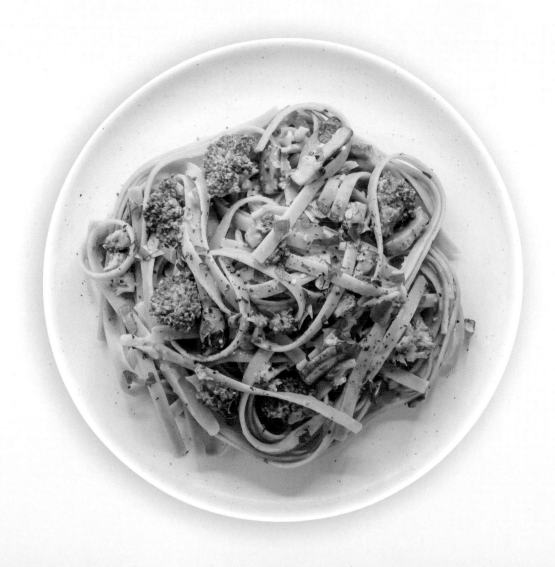

creamy mushroom pasta

With a rich, velvety cashew sauce, this is truly a to-die-for dish. The best part? You can have it on the table in less than twenty minutes. It's as simple as cooking the pasta, blending the sauce, and putting it all together in a big skillet. I love to top mine with fresh parsley and a squeeze of lemon juice.

MAKES 4 servings   ✦   **FROM START TO FINISH:** 20 minutes

1 (17-ounce) package whole wheat rigatoni pasta

1 cup cashews, soaked in water overnight or boiled for 15 minutes

1 teaspoon paprika

4 garlic cloves, peeled

1 cup unsweetened almond milk

1 teaspoon freshly squeezed lemon juice

1 teaspoon salt, plus more to serve

3 cups cremini mushrooms, roughly chopped

1 cup fresh basil or spinach

Freshly ground black pepper, to serve

Red pepper flakes, to serve

Chopped fresh herbs, to serve (optional)

1. Cook the pasta according to the package directions until al dente, reserving ½ cup of pasta water before draining.

2. **Meanwhile, make the sauce:** Combine the cashews, paprika, garlic, almond milk, lemon juice, and salt in a blender and blend until smooth.

3. Combine the mushrooms with 1 to 2 tablespoons of water in a large skillet, and panfry over medium heat until softened, about 3 minutes.

4. Pour the sauce into the skillet along with the rigatoni, reserved pasta water, and basil and stir until combined. Season with salt, black pepper, and red pepper flakes as desired.

notes

For a gluten-free version, use a brown rice or chickpea pasta instead.

For a nut-free version, use soaked sunflower seeds instead of the almond milk.

RIGATONI

CASHEWS

PAPRIKA

GARLIC (CLOVES)

ALMOND MILK

LEMON (JUICE)

CREMINI MUSHROOMS

BASIL (FRESH)

RED PEPPER FLAKES

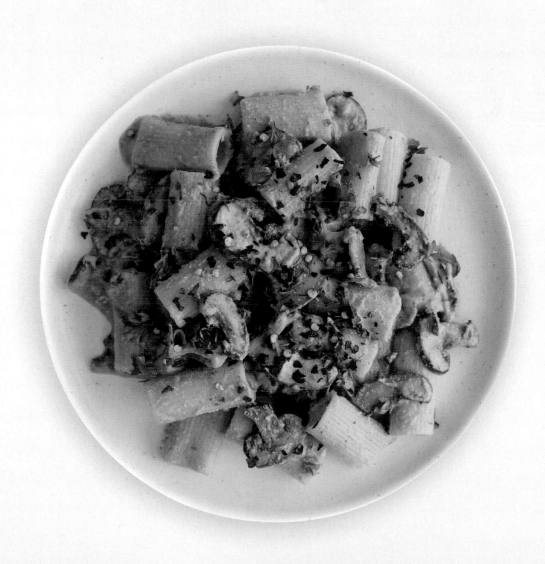

garden bolognese

Of any recipe in this cookbook, I'd love for you to try this simple plant-filled Bolognese. It is perhaps my favorite dish and comes together effortlessly. The best part about it is that the meaty texture of the sauce is made entirely of plants, producing a fiber- and nutrient-rich sauce perfect for topping just about any pasta dish.

MAKES 4 servings ✦ **FROM START TO FINISH:** 35 minutes

1 (16-ounce) package whole-grain fettuccine

4 garlic cloves, peeled and minced

1 yellow onion

2 red bell peppers

2 cups cremini mushrooms

1½ cups cherry tomatoes

3 cups spinach

2 tablespoons balsamic vinegar

1 (24-ounce) jar vegan pasta sauce (about 3 cups)

½ teaspoon red pepper flakes

1 cup basil

Freshly ground black pepper, to serve

1. Cook the pasta according to the package directions.

2. Combine the garlic with 1 to 2 tablespoons of water in a skillet with a lid (you'll need it later), and sauté over medium heat until fragrant, about 2 minutes.

3. Meanwhile, slice the onion into four pieces and place in a food processor. Mince, then add to the skillet and sauté for 3 to 5 minutes, or until softened.

4. Slice the bell peppers into large chunks and place in the food processor. Mince, then incorporate into the mixture in the skillet.

5. Working one vegetable at a time, repeat the same step with your mushrooms, cherry tomatoes, and spinach, until you have a large veggie mince sautéing over medium heat.

6. Next, add the balsamic vinegar and sauté for 4 to 5 minutes until all the vegetables are incorporated.

7. Finally, add the pasta sauce, red pepper flakes, and basil. Stir until completely combined, bring to a boil, then cover and simmer for 10 minutes.

8. Enjoy over a bed of the freshly cooked whole-grain fettuccine, sprinkled with black pepper.

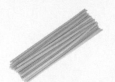

FETTUCCINE **GARLIC (CLOVES)** **YELLOW ONION** **RED BELL PEPPER** **CREMINI MUSHROOMS** **CHERRY TOMATOES**

SPINACH **BALSAMIC VINEGAR** **PASTA SAUCE** **RED PEPPER FLAKES** **BASIL (FRESH)**

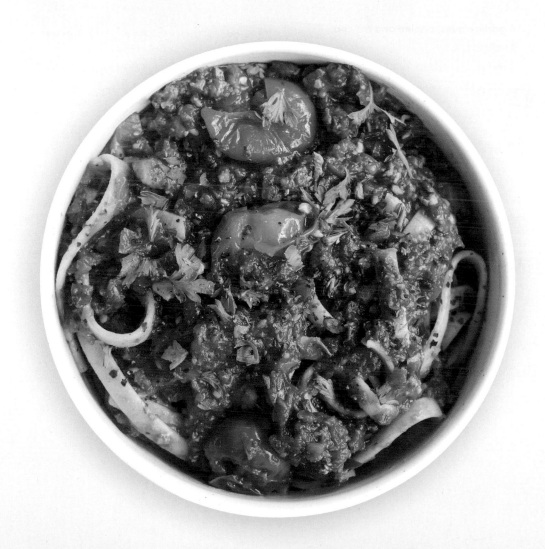

ginger garlic noodz

Ginger and garlic together are a match made in heaven. Not only do they add incredible flavor and aroma to recipes like this noodle dish, they both have amazing health-promoting properties, such as warding off the common cold, reducing inflammation, and aiding digestion.

MAKES 4 servings ✦ **FROM START TO FINISH:** 25 minutes

7 ounces uncooked brown rice vermicelli noodles

1 (1-inch-long) piece fresh ginger, peeled and minced

6 garlic cloves, peeled and minced

2 cups shredded green cabbage (about 14 ounces)

1 medium-size yellow onion, sliced

2 tablespoons cornstarch + 2 tablespoons warm water

2 tablespoons cider vinegar

½ cup vegetable broth

2 tablespoons tamari or soy sauce

1½ cups oyster mushrooms, sliced

1 cup sugar snap peas

¼ cup black sesame seeds

3 hot chile peppers (optional)

1. Cook the noodles according to the package directions and set aside.

2. Meanwhile, heat a large skillet over medium heat, and add 1 to 2 tablespoons of water along with the minced ginger and garlic. Stir-fry until fragrant, about 1 minute.

3. Add the cabbage and onion to the skillet and stir-fry until softened, 3 to 5 minutes.

4. Create a cornstarch slurry by combining the cornstarch and warm water in a small bowl. Set aside.

5. Now, add the cider vinegar, vegetable broth, tamari, oyster mushrooms, and snap peas to the skillet. Bring the liquid to a boil, then add the cornstarch slurry to thicken.

6. Add the noodles and stir-fry for 30 seconds until everything is combined and heated through, about 2 minutes.

7. Serve with sesame seeds sprinkled over the top and chile peppers, as desired.

note For a gluten-free version, use wheat-free tamari, not soy sauce.

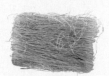

BROWN RICE VERMICELLI NOODLES **GINGER (FRESH)** **GARLIC (CLOVES)** **GREEN CABBAGE** **YELLOW ONION**

CORNSTARCH **CIDER VINEGAR** **VEGETABLE BROTH** **TAMARI**

   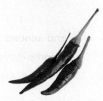

OYSTER MUSHROOMS **SNAP PEAS** **SESAME SEEDS (BLACK)** **CHILE PEPPERS (OPTIONAL)**

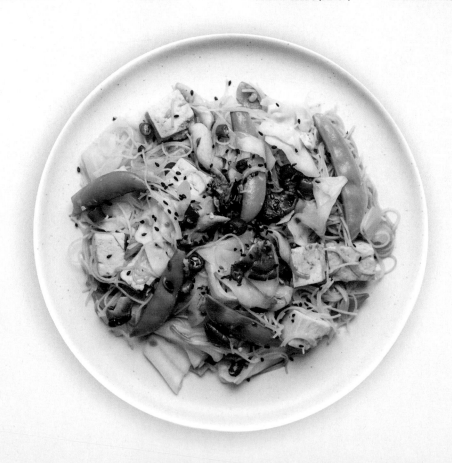

sheet pan fajitas

You'll be shocked at how simple these sheet pan fajitas are to whip together, and the cleanup is minimal. Throw all your veggies and spices on a pan, roast for twenty-five minutes, and serve on your preferred tortillas with toppings of choice. This is a perfect kid- or crowd-pleasing meal.

MAKES 4 servings, 2 fajitas per serving ✦ **FROM START TO FINISH:** 35 minutes

2 portobello mushroom caps, sliced into strips

2 red bell peppers, seeded and sliced into strips

1½ medium-size yellow onions, sliced into strips

½ teaspoon salt

1 teaspoon chili powder

½ teaspoon garlic powder

½ teaspoon ground cumin

¼ cup fresh cilantro, chopped

8 corn tortillas

OPTIONAL TOPPINGS
Avocado

Coconut yogurt

Salsa

1. Preheat the oven to 400°F and line a baking sheet with parchment paper.

2. Toss together the portobello strips, bell peppers, onions, salt, chili powder, garlic powder, cumin, and cilantro in a bowl. Pour onto the baking sheet and spread out evenly. Roast for 25 minutes, tossing halfway through.

3. If desired, you can warm the tortillas by wrapping a stack of them in foil and heating them in a 350°F oven for 15 to 20 minutes.

4. Divide the portobello mixture among the tortillas, and top with avocado, coconut yogurt (as a sour cream replacement), and salsa, as desired.

PORTOBELLO

RED BELL PEPPER

YELLOW ONION

CHILI POWDER

GARLIC POWDER

CUMIN

CILANTRO

CORN TORTILLA

AVOCADO (OPTIONAL)

COCONUT YOGURT (OPTIONAL)

SALSA (OPTIONAL)

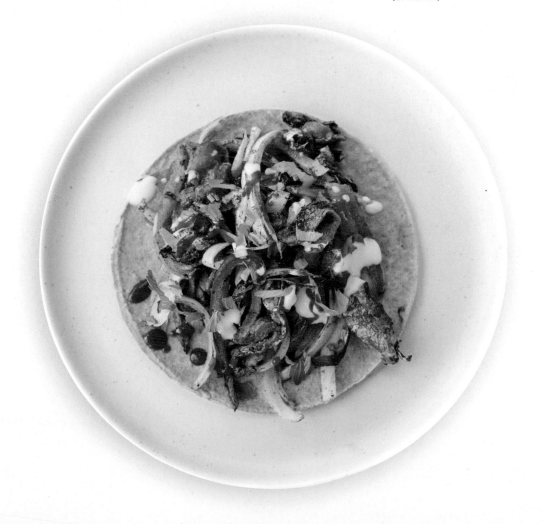

the big boss burrito

For these burritos, try to find the largest tortilla wraps available (I used 12-inch)! This is essential to pack in all the amazing plant-based ingredients, such as black beans, rice, sautéed vegetables, and let's not forget the avocado. For best results, throw the wrapped burrito on a grill or heat in a pan to seal and get the outside a bit crunchy and all the ingredients melty on the inside.

MAKES 4 servings ✦ **FROM START TO FINISH:** 30 minutes

2 red bell peppers, seeded and chopped

1 medium-size yellow onion, chopped

1½ cups cremini mushrooms

½ teaspoon chili powder

½ teaspoon ground cumin

½ teaspoon garlic powder

½ teaspoon salt

4 large whole wheat tortillas

2 cups cooked brown rice

1 (15-ounce) can black beans (about 1½ cups), drained and rinsed

1 cup shredded iceberg lettuce

2 avocados, peeled, pitted, and mashed

¼ cup salsa

¼ cup coconut yogurt

Hot sauce (optional)

1. Combine the bell peppers, onions, mushrooms, chili powder, cumin, garlic powder, and salt with 1 to 2 tablespoons of water in a large skillet and sauté over medium heat until softened, 5 to 8 minutes.

2. **Prepare the burritos:** Lay a tortilla flat on a plate. Add ¼ cup of the rice to the center of the tortilla, followed by the black beans, sautéed vegetables, and shredded lettuce. Top with avocado, salsa, coconut yogurt, and hot sauce, if desired. Fold in the sides and tightly roll.

3. To seal, place a burrito, seam side down, on barbecue grill or skillet that has been heated to medium or high heat. Cook for 3 to 5 minutes, or until golden brown, then flip and repeat on the other side.

notes

There are endless ways to customize these burritos. Swap out black beans for pinto beans or chopped tofu, add pico de gallo instead of salsa, omit the mushrooms, use spinach instead of lettuce, and so on.

For a gluten-free version, omit the tortilla and serve the burrito toppings over rice instead.

RED BELL PEPPER

YELLOW ONION

CREMINI MUSHROOMS

CHILI POWDER

CUMIN

GARLIC POWDER

WHOLE WHEAT TORTILLA

BROWN RICE

BLACK BEANS

LETTUCE

AVOCADO

SALSA

COCONUT YOGURT

HOT SAUCE (OPTIONAL)

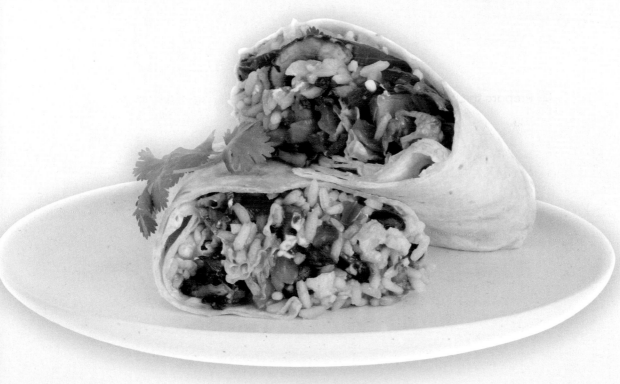

10-minute tacos

For a recipe that comes together in a mere ten minutes, these tacos are truly phenomenal. To make a realistic taco meat, I combine walnuts and mushrooms with chili powder and cumin in a food processor, then sauté to soften. Serve in a corn tortilla for taco night, or in a salad, burrito, or bowl if preferred.

MAKES 4 servings (2 tacos per serving) ✦ **FROM START TO FINISH:** 10 minutes

½ cup + 2 tablespoons walnuts

2 cups mushrooms

2 teaspoons cider vinegar

2½ tablespoons tamari or soy sauce

1¼ teaspoons ground cumin

¾ teaspoon chili powder

8 corn tortillas

SUGGESTED TOPPINGS

1 avocado, peeled, pitted, and mashed

1 red onion, chopped

1 tomato, chopped

½ cup Vegan Queso (page 214)

½ cup coconut yogurt

Fresh cilantro (optional)

1. Combine the walnuts, mushrooms, cider vinegar, tamari, and spices in a food processor. Process until a chunky, thick texture is achieved.

2. Place the walnut mixture in a skillet and sauté over medium heat until softened, 6 to 8 minutes.

3. Add the walnut mixture to the corn tortillas as well as your preferred toppings, such as avocado, red onion, tomato, Vegan Queso, and coconut yogurt. Garnish with fresh cilantro as desired.

notes

For a nut-free version, use cauliflower instead of walnuts in the same amount.

For a gluten-free version, use wheat-free tamari, not soy sauce.

WALNUTS

MUSHROOMS

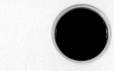

CIDER VINEGAR

TAMARI

CUMIN

CHILI POWDER

CORN TORTILLAS

AVOCADO

RED ONION

TOMATO

VEGAN QUESO

COCONUT YOGURT

CILANTRO (OPTIONAL)

the main event

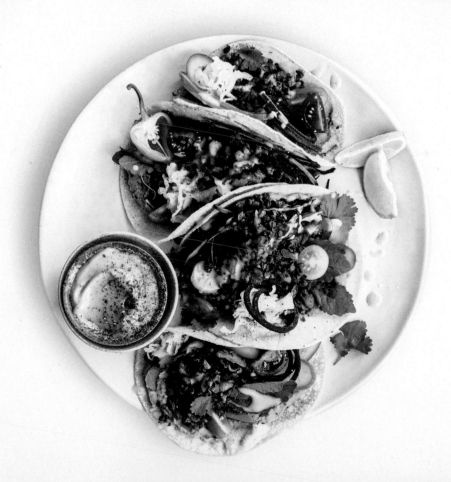

rainbow summer rolls

These rolls scream "sunshine," and they're one of my favorite light and fresh weeknight meals. Rolling fresh rice paper wraps for the first time can be a challenge, but once you've done one or two, you'll get the hang of it. For greens, I've opted for kale in this recipe, which provides a nice crunch and slight bitter note, but you could also use basil or mint if you'd prefer!

MAKES 4 servings (4 rolls per serving)   ✦   **FROM START TO FINISH:** 20 minutes

12 edible rice paper sheets

1 cup cooked brown rice vermicelli noodles (about 2 ounces dried)

1 carrot, peeled and sliced into thin matchsticks

1 cup baby kale, massaged and chopped

1 red bell pepper, seeded and sliced

½ cucumber, sliced into matchsticks

1 cup roughly chopped purple cabbage

2 tablespoons black sesame seeds

Spicy Peanut Dressing (page 203) or low-sodium tamari, to serve

1. **Prepare the rice paper:** Pour very hot water into a shallow dish and immerse the rice paper sheets for 10 to 15 seconds, just to soften. Carefully transfer to a cutting board.

2. Add a small portion of the noodles, carrots, kale, bell pepper, cucumber, cabbage, and sesame seeds to a rice paper sheet. Gently fold over once, tuck in the edges, then continue rolling until the seam is sealed.

3. Place, seam side down, on a serving platter. Repeat until all the fillings are used up. Serve with peanut dressing or low-sodium tamari.

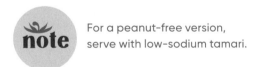

note For a peanut-free version, serve with low-sodium tamari.

RICE PAPER

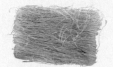

BROWN RICE VERMICELLI NOODLES

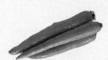

CARROT

KALE

RED BELL PEPPER

CUCUMBER

PURPLE CABBAGE

SESAME SEEDS (BLACK)

SPICY PEANUT DRESSING

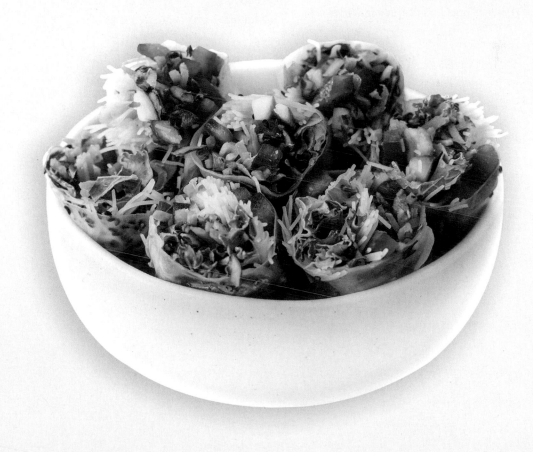

staple tempeh stir-fry

I make a version of this stir-fry at least once a week. The beauty of it is, you can use up basically any vegetable you have lying around in your fridge and it will still taste delicious. To give a sweet and salty flavor, we love using hoisin sauce, but in a pinch you could use pure maple syrup or your favorite vegan sweetener instead. For the purpose of this recipe, I've served it with basmati rice, but you could use vermicelli noodles or lettuce wraps instead.

MAKES 4 servings ✦ **FROM START TO FINISH:** 25 minutes

1 cup uncooked basmati rice

SAUCE
1 (½-inch-long) piece fresh ginger, peeled and minced

1 tablespoon cider vinegar

¼ cup tamari or soy sauce

3 tablespoons hoisin sauce

¼ cup vegetable broth

1 tablespoon cornstarch

STIR-FRY
4 garlic cloves, minced

1 medium-size yellow onion, sliced

1 (8-ounce) package tempeh, sliced into bite-size pieces

2 red bell peppers, seeded and sliced

2 carrots, ribboned

1½ cups cremini mushrooms, chopped

2 tablespoons sesame seeds

1. Cook the rice according to the package directions.

2. **Make the stir-fry sauce:** Combine the ginger, cider vinegar, tamari, hoisin sauce, vegetable broth, and cornstarch in a bowl. Whisk or blend until completely combined.

3. Meanwhile, in a pan over medium heat, combine the garlic and onion with 2 tablespoons of water in a large skillet. Sauté until the onion becomes translucent, about 5 minutes.

4. Add the sliced tempeh and bell peppers to the skillet. Cook for about 5 minutes, or until the tempeh begins to brown.

5. Next, add your stir-fry sauce, carrots, and mushrooms. Stir until completely combined and cook for an additional 3 to 5 minutes, or until softened.

6. Serve over the cooked rice and garnish with sesame seeds.

note For a gluten-free version, use gluten-free hoisin sauce.

BASMATI RICE

 GINGER (FRESH)

 CIDER VINEGAR

 TAMARI

 HOISIN SAUCE

 VEGETABLE BROTH

 CORNSTARCH

 GARLIC (CLOVES)

 YELLOW ONION

 TEMPEH

 RED BELL PEPPER

 CARROTS

 CREMINI MUSHROOMS

 SESAME SEEDS

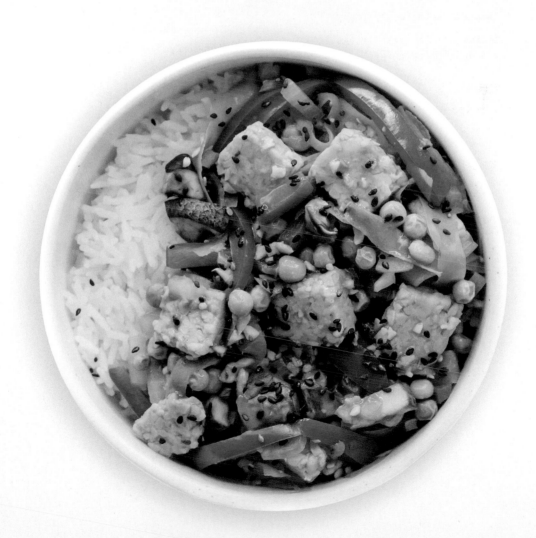

simple peanut sauce stir-fry

When in doubt, throw a bunch of vegetables in a pan and pour on this savory to-die-for peanut sauce! This quick and delicious plant-based dish comes together in less than twenty-five minutes and will be your new favorite weeknight meal.

MAKES 4 servings ✦ **FROM START TO FINISH:** 25 minutes

1 cup uncooked basmati rice

SAUCE
½ cup warm water

3 tablespoons peanut butter

3 tablespoons hoisin sauce

2 tablespoons tamari or soy sauce

1 tablespoon cornstarch

STIR-FRY
1 (16-ounce) package extra-firm tofu, pressed and chopped into 1-inch cubes

1½ cups sugar snap peas

1 red bell pepper, seeded and sliced

½ medium-size yellow onion, diced

1 carrot, peeled and ribboned

Juice of 1 lime

Crushed peanuts, to serve

1. Cook the rice according to the package directions.

2. **Prepare the peanut sauce:** Combine the water, peanut butter, hoisin sauce, tamari, and cornstarch in a bowl. Whisk until smooth.

3. **Prepare the stir-fry:** Place the tofu cubes in a large skillet with 3 tablespoons of water. Sauté over medium heat, adding more water if needed, until the tofu is browned slightly, 5 to 7 minutes.

4. Add the sugar snap peas, bell pepper, onion, and carrot to the skillet with an additional ¼ cup of water. Sauté until the vegetables have softened slightly, 3 to 4 minutes.

5. Finally, pour in the peanut sauce and stir for 1 more minute before turning off the heat.

6. Serve over the rice with fresh lime juice and crushed peanuts, as desired.

notes

For a peanut-free version, use a soy-based peanut butter alternative or sunflower seed butter in place of peanut butter.

For a gluten-free version, use wheat-free tamari.

BASMATI RICE

 PEANUT BUTTER

 HOISIN SAUCE

 TAMARI

 CORNSTARCH

 EXTRA-FIRM TOFU

 SNAP PEAS

 RED BELL PEPPER

 YELLOW ONION

 CARROT

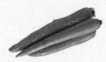 LIME (JUICE)

 PEANUTS

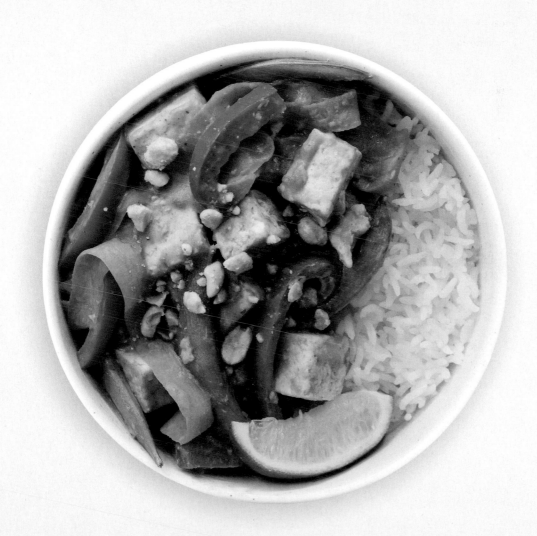

plant-packed pad thai

When my fiancé, Jesse, and I traveled to Thailand in 2017, we were fortunate to take an authentic cooking class in a beachside town called Krabi. One of the dishes we assembled was pad Thai, and the cooking instructor was generous in guiding me on some vegan substitutions during the class. This recipe is loosely based on authentic pad Thai, including traditional tamarind paste, with the addition of several vegetables and plant-based ingredient substitutions.

MAKES 4 servings ✦ **FROM START TO FINISH:** 35 minutes

1 (16-ounce) package (⅛- to ¼-inch-wide) rice noodles

SAUCE

¼ cup tamari or soy sauce

2½ tablespoons coconut sugar or pure maple syrup

6 tablespoons warm water

3 tablespoons tamarind paste or rice vinegar

TOFU EGG

10 ounces extra-firm tofu

½ teaspoon black salt (kala namak)

½ teaspoon ground turmeric

STIR-FRIED VEGETABLES

4 garlic cloves, peeled and minced

1 red onion, diced

2 carrots, ribboned

TO SERVE

½ bunch green onions, chopped

¼ cup crushed peanuts

½ cup fresh cilantro, chopped

Freshly squeezed lime juice, as desired

Red pepper flakes

1. Cook the rice noodles according to the package directions.

2. **Prepare the sauce:** Whisk together the tamari, coconut sugar, warm water, and tamarind paste in a small bowl until combined. Set aside.

3. **Prepare the tofu egg:** Place the tofu on a cutting board or plate, and mash it with the back of a fork. Combine the tofu, black salt, and turmeric in a large skillet and sauté over medium heat until cooked, about 5 minutes. Pour the tofu back onto the plate and set aside.

4. **Prepare the stir-fry:** In the same skillet, combine the garlic, red onion, and carrots with a tablespoon of water, if needed, and sauté over medium heat for 2 minutes, or until softened slightly.

5. Next, add the cooked rice noodles and the sauce and gently stir until combined, followed by the tofu egg. Plate and garnish with green onions, crushed peanuts, cilantro, lime juice, and red pepper flakes, as desired.

RICE NOODLES

TAMARI

COCONUT SUGAR

TAMARIND PASTE

EXTRA-FIRM TOFU

KALA NAMAK
(BLACK SALT)

TURMERIC

GARLIC (CLOVES)

RED ONION

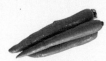
CARROTS

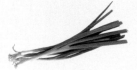
GREEN ONION

PEANUTS

CILANTRO

LIME (JUICE)

RED PEPPER FLAKES

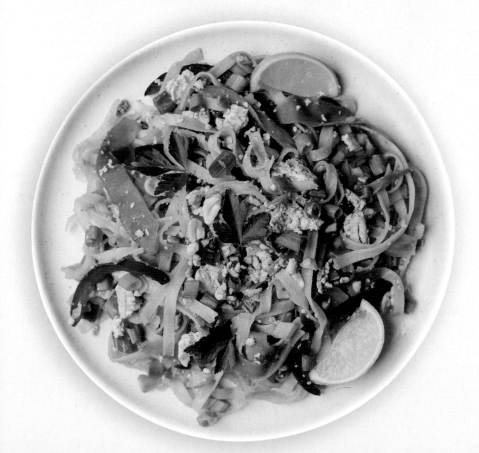

notes

For a gluten-
free version,
use wheat-free
tamari, not soy
sauce.

For a peanut-
free version, omit
the peanuts.

pineapple cauliflower fried rice

Cauliflower has to be the most versatile food on the planet, and it makes an amazing rice substitute! You can generally find it at most grocery stores already ground into "rice," or simply throw your florets in a food processor to get a rice consistency. To jazz up this cauliflower fried rice, I serve it up with chopped pineapple, which provides the perfect tang. For a fancy serving option, use fresh pineapple for the recipe, then hollow out the halves!

MAKES 4 servings ✦ **FROM START TO FINISH:** 20 minutes

1½ cups chopped pineapple

¼ cup vegetable broth

3 garlic cloves, peeled and minced

1 red onion, diced

4 carrots, diced

8 cups cauliflower rice (about 1 medium-size head, grated in a food processor)

1½ cups frozen peas

4 green onions, diced

1 cup cremini mushrooms, chopped

⅓ cup tamari or soy sauce

Salt and freshly ground black pepper

1. If making pineapple serving bowls, slice each pineapple in half and hollow out both halves to create four bowls, reserving 1½ cups of the pineapple to add to the fried rice.

2. Heat the vegetable broth in a large skillet over medium-high heat. Add the garlic and red onion and sauté until fragrant, about 1 minute. Add the carrots and continue to cook until softened, 3 to 5 minutes.

3. Add the riced cauliflower, peas, green onions, mushrooms, tamari, and salt and pepper to taste.

4. Cook, stirring frequently, for about 10 minutes, or until the cauliflower is tender. At the end, add the chunks of pineapple and stir until combined.

5. Divide and transfer into the hollowed-out pineapples.

note For a gluten-free version, use wheat-free tamari, not soy sauce.

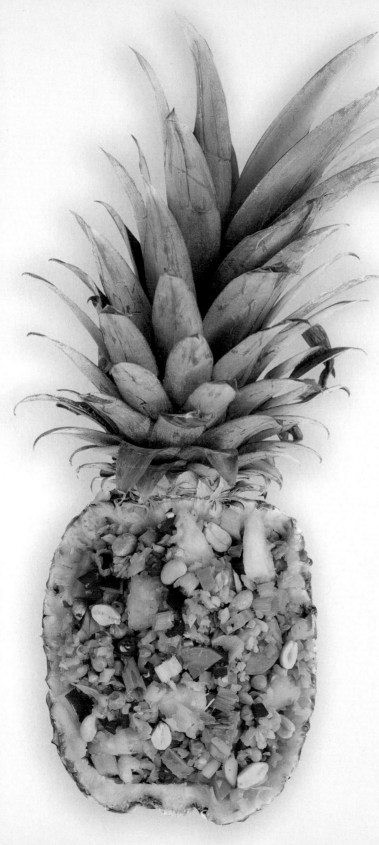

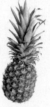

PINEAPPLE

VEGETABLE BROTH

GARLIC (CLOVES)

RED ONION

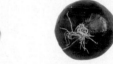

CARROTS

CAULIFLOWER RICE

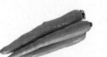

GREEN PEAS

GREEN ONIONS

CREMINI MUSHROOMS

TAMARI

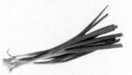

hoisin broccoli spicy rice

This recipe goes out to all my spice lovers! I'm a spice fanatic, and would add hot red chile peppers to just about any dish if I could. My fiancé, on the other hand, despises spicy food, so I make this dish whenever he's out of town. If you want to try this dish but can't handle the heat, simply omit the red chile peppers.

MAKES 4 servings ✦ **FROM START TO FINISH:** 25 minutes

1 cup uncooked jasmine rice

1 head broccoli, chopped into florets

3 red chile peppers, diced

½ red onion, diced

3 garlic cloves, peeled and minced

2 tablespoons cider vinegar

3½ tablespoons hoisin sauce

1 teaspoon tamari or soy sauce

1. Cook the rice according to the package directions.

2. Combine the broccoli, chile peppers, red onion, garlic, and cider vinegar in a large skillet and sauté over medium heat until softened and slightly charred, about 5 minutes, adding a tablespoon of water or as needed.

3. Stir in the hoisin sauce and tamari and allow to glaze for a minute. Next, add the rice and stir until everything is combined.

note For a gluten-free version, use gluten-free hoisin sauce and also wheat-free tamari, not soy sauce.

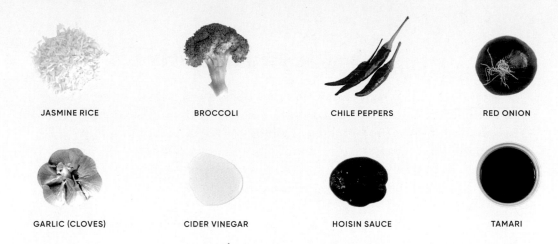

JASMINE RICE · BROCCOLI · CHILE PEPPERS · RED ONION

GARLIC (CLOVES) · CIDER VINEGAR · HOISIN SAUCE · TAMARI

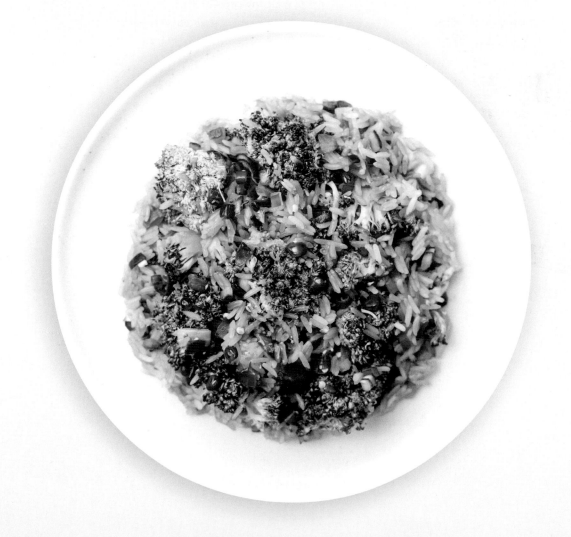

sweet 'n' spicy tofu skewers

These tofu skewers are the perfect recipe to have on hand if you're heading to a summer barbecue and aren't sure whether there will be any veggie options. The tofu is quickly marinated in a delicious blend of sriracha, tamari, and maple syrup, then placed on skewers with beaming summer vegetables like red onion and zucchini. You can use reusable stainless steel skewers or bamboo skewers, as desired. I love to serve these over a bed of rice, or as the topping on a salad.

MAKES 4 servings (about 12 skewers, 3 skewers per person)

FROM START TO FINISH: 30 minutes

2 teaspoons sriracha

½ cup tamari or soy sauce

2 tablespoons pure maple syrup

2 tablespoons cider vinegar

1 (16-ounce) package extra-firm tofu, pressed, sliced into 1-inch cubes

1 red bell pepper, seeded and chopped into 1-inch pieces

1 red onion, sliced into 1-inch pieces

1 cup white mushrooms, sliced into 1-inch pieces

1 medium-size zucchini, sliced into 1-inch pieces

1. Whisk together the sriracha, tamari, maple syrup, and cider vinegar in a bowl. Put the tofu in the bowl and stir around until the marinade has coated both sides. Place in the fridge to marinate for 15 minutes, stirring halfway through.

2. Preheat a grill to between 400° and 450°F.

3. Assemble the skewers, alternating between the tofu and vegetables.

4. Grill the skewers for 5 minutes on each side, or until browned slightly. Alternatively, fry the skewers in a skillet over medium heat, with a tablespoon of water or as needed, until browned on each side. Serve immediately.

notes

For a gluten-free version, use wheat-free tamari, not soy sauce.

If using bamboo skewers, to prevent burning, soak them for at least 30 minutes in water before using.

sweet 'n' spicy tofu skewers

These tofu skewers are the perfect recipe to have on hand if you're heading to a summer barbecue and aren't sure whether there will be any veggie options. The tofu is quickly marinated in a delicious blend of sriracha, tamari, and maple syrup, then placed on skewers with beaming summer vegetables like red onion and zucchini. You can use reusable stainless steel skewers or bamboo skewers, as desired. I love to serve these over a bed of rice, or as the topping on a salad.

MAKES 4 servings (about 12 skewers, 3 skewers per person)
FROM START TO FINISH: 30 minutes

2 teaspoons sriracha

½ cup tamari or soy sauce

2 tablespoons pure maple syrup

2 tablespoons cider vinegar

1 (16-ounce) package extra-firm tofu, pressed, sliced into 1-inch cubes

1 red bell pepper, seeded and chopped into 1-inch pieces

1 red onion, sliced into 1-inch pieces

1 cup white mushrooms, sliced into 1-inch pieces

1 medium-size zucchini, sliced into 1-inch pieces

1. Whisk together the sriracha, tamari, maple syrup, and cider vinegar in a bowl. Put the tofu in the bowl and stir around until the marinade has coated both sides. Place in the fridge to marinate for 15 minutes, stirring halfway through.

2. Preheat a grill to between 400° and 450°F.

3. Assemble the skewers, alternating between the tofu and vegetables.

4. Grill the skewers for 5 minutes on each side, or until browned slightly. Alternatively, fry the skewers in a skillet over medium heat, with a tablespoon of water or as needed, until browned on each side. Serve immediately.

notes

For a gluten-free version, use wheat-free tamari, not soy sauce.

If using bamboo skewers, to prevent burning, soak them for at least 30 minutes in water before using.

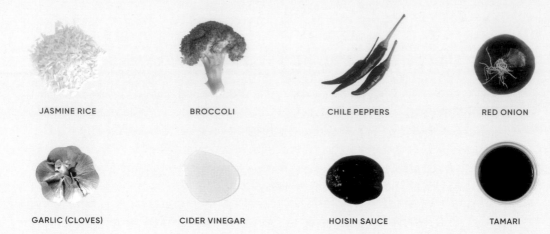

JASMINE RICE   BROCCOLI   CHILE PEPPERS   RED ONION

GARLIC (CLOVES)   CIDER VINEGAR   HOISIN SAUCE   TAMARI

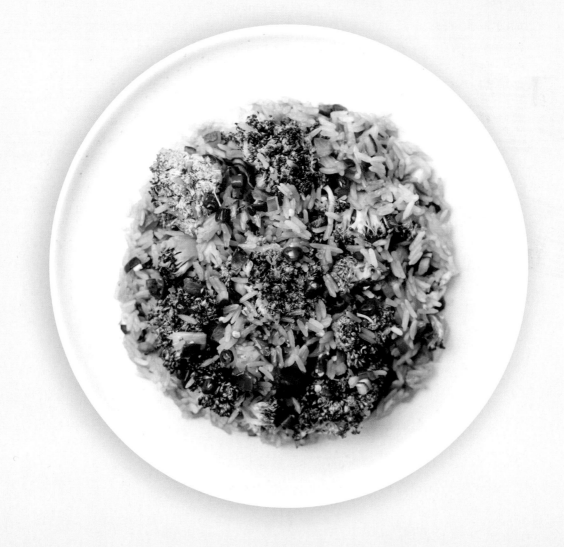

SRIRACHA

TAMARI

MAPLE SYRUP

CIDER VINEGAR

EXTRA-FIRM TOFU

RED BELL PEPPER

RED ONION

WHITE MUSHROOMS

ZUCCHINI

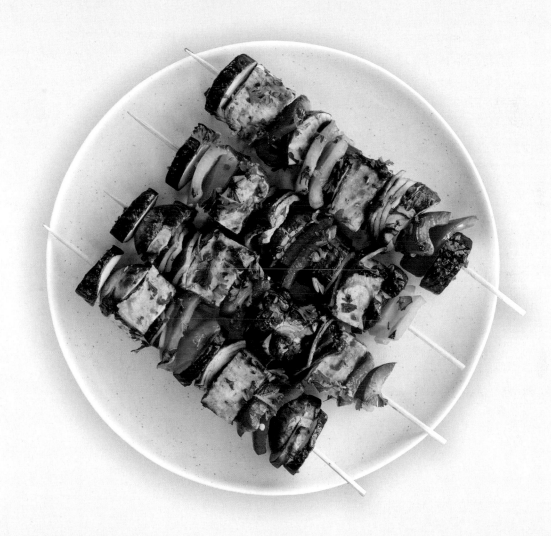

"butter" chickpeas

This thick, fragrant stew spiced with curry powder, cumin, and paprika is loosely inspired by Indian butter chicken. It's made rich and velvety with the addition of almond butter and canned coconut milk. You could enjoy this with chunks of extra-firm tofu, or the addition of your favorite vegetables, such as bell pepper and potato.

MAKES 4 servings (about 1¼ cups of curry and ¾ cup of rice per serving)
FROM START TO FINISH: 25 minutes

1 cup uncooked basmati rice

1 medium-size yellow onion, chopped

3 garlic cloves, peeled and minced

2½ teaspoons curry powder

2 teaspoons ground cumin

½ teaspoon paprika

1 (15-ounce) can crushed tomatoes (about 1½ cups), with juices

1 (15-ounce) can chickpeas (about 1½ cups), drained and rinsed

¾ cup canned full-fat or light coconut milk

¼ cup unsweetened almond butter

1 tablespoon cider vinegar

1 teaspoon pure maple syrup

1 tablespoon tamari or soy sauce

¼ cup fresh cilantro

1. Cook the rice according to the package directions.

2. Combine the onion, garlic, and 1 to 2 tablespoons of water in a large skillet with a lid (you'll need it later). Sauté over medium heat until the onion is translucent, about 3 minutes.

3. Add the curry powder, cumin, and paprika and stir until the onion mixture is covered.

4. Now, add the crushed tomatoes, chickpeas, coconut milk, and almond butter.

5. Stir in the cider vinegar, maple syrup, and tamari, tasting and adjusting the sweet and salty flavors as desired.

6. Cover and simmer for 10 minutes. Serve over the rice with fresh cilantro.

 note For a nut-free version, use a soy-based peanut butter substitute or tahini in place of almond butter.

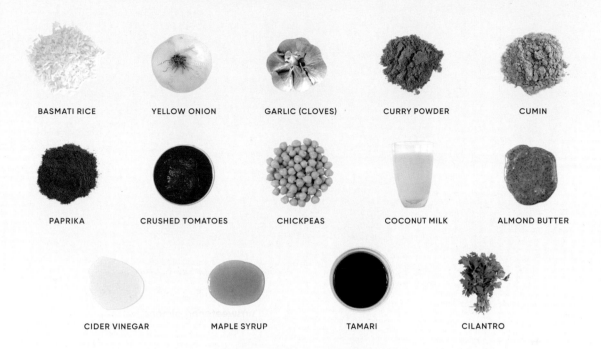

BASMATI RICE

YELLOW ONION

GARLIC (CLOVES)

CURRY POWDER

CUMIN

PAPRIKA

CRUSHED TOMATOES

CHICKPEAS

COCONUT MILK

ALMOND BUTTER

CIDER VINEGAR

MAPLE SYRUP

TAMARI

CILANTRO

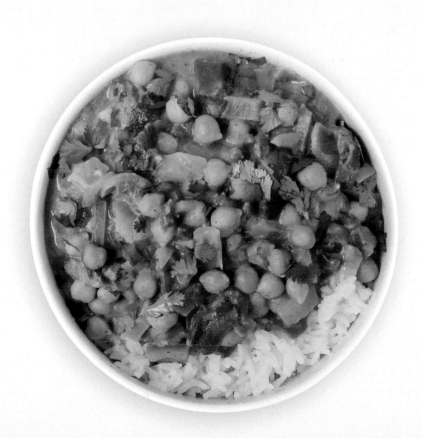

"everything but the kitchen sink" curry

This savory and fragrant curry is loosely inspired by Tikka Masala, an Indian dish that typically sees chunks of roasted marinated chicken in a beautifully spiced gravy. Instead of using chicken, this curry is packed to the brim with sweet potato, cauliflower, and green peas, but really it will work with just about any vegetable you have on hand.

MAKES 4 servings (about 1¾ cups of curry per serving) ✦ **FROM START TO FINISH:** 30 minutes

1 cup uncooked basmati rice

¼ cup vegetable broth

1 medium-size sweet potato, unpeeled, chopped into small cubes

1 medium-size yellow onion, diced

6 garlic cloves, peeled and minced

1 small head cauliflower, chopped into florets

1 red bell pepper, seeded and sliced

2 tablespoons garam masala

1 teaspoon ground ginger

1 teaspoon ground turmeric

1½ teaspoons ground cinnamon, Ceylon if possible

1 teaspoon sea salt

1 (15-ounce) can full-fat or light coconut milk (about 1½ cups)

1 (15-ounce) can crushed tomatoes (about 1½ cups), including liquid

1 tablespoon pure maple syrup

1½ cups frozen green peas

1½ cups curly kale, chopped

1. Cook the rice according to the package directions.

2. Meanwhile, heat the vegetable broth in a large skillet with a lid (you'll need it later) over medium heat. Add the sweet potato, onion, and garlic. Sauté until the sweet potato has softened slightly, 6 and 8 minutes.

3. Add the cauliflower florets and bell pepper to the pot, along with the garam masala, ginger, turmeric, cinnamon, and salt. Stir until the vegetables are coated with the spices and the dish becomes fragrant, 2 to 3 minutes.

4. Add the coconut milk, crushed tomatoes, and maple syrup to the pot. Stir until combined, bring to a boil and then simmer, covered, over low heat until the sweet potatoes and cauliflower are fork-tender, about 12 minutes.

5. Taste and adjust the seasonings as needed. Add the green peas and kale and stir until they have respectively thawed and wilted.

6. Enjoy served over the rice.

BASMATI RICE

VEGETABLE BROTH

SWEET POTATO

YELLOW ONION

GARLIC (CLOVES)

CAULIFLOWER

RED BELL PEPPER

GARAM MASALA

GINGER SPICE

TURMERIC

CINNAMON

COCONUT MILK

CRUSHED TOMATOES

MAPLE SYRUP

GREEN PEAS

KALE

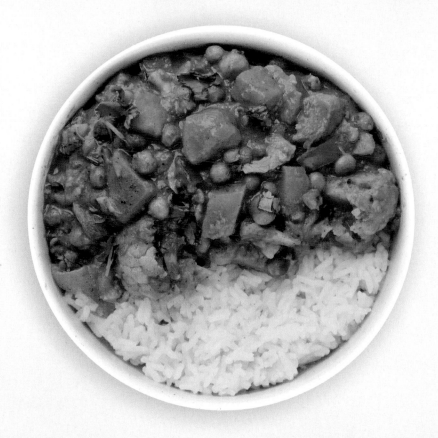

note

This is fantastic with extra-firm tofu, shredded Brussels sprouts, tofu, and more.

"can't believe it's vegan" lasagna

Kids, picky eaters, and meat lovers will never know this hearty lasagna is packed with vegetables. The secret is throwing the veggies in the food processor so they create a meaty consistency in the sauce. When added to your favorite pasta sauce, then layered with lasagna noodles and my creamy Tofu Ricotta (page 215), this is truly a to-die-for meal perfect for serving guests.

MAKES 6 servings ✦ **FROM START TO FINISH:** 50 minutes

2 cups spinach

1 red bell pepper, seeded and quartered

1 medium-size yellow onion, peeled and quartered

1½ cups cremini mushrooms

4 garlic cloves, peeled

2 (24-ounce) jars vegan pasta sauce of your choice (about 6 cups)

1 (12-ounce) package oven-ready brown rice or whole wheat lasagna noodles

6 servings Tofu Ricotta (page 215)

1. Preheat the oven to 350°F.

2. **Prepare the vegetable sauce:** Place the spinach, red bell pepper, yellow onion, cremini mushrooms, and garlic in a food processor one at a time, pulsing between each addition until finely ground. Transfer the ground vegetables to a large skillet and sauté over medium heat until they become fragrant and soft, for about 5 minutes.

3. Add the two jars of pasta sauce to the veggie mixture and stir until completely combined. Bring to a boil, then simmer over low heat for 5 minutes.

4. To assemble the lasagna, pour a generous 1-cup serving of the vegetable sauce into the bottom of a 9 x 13-inch casserole dish or baking pan.

5. Next, add three of the lasagna noodles, according to the package directions. Top with another generous serving of sauce, then spread one-quarter of the vegan ricotta on top, using a spatula. Repeat these steps until all the noodles are used up.

6. Once you reach the end, pour the remaining sauce over the top layer of lasagna and place blobs of the ricotta mixture on top.

7. Cover tightly with foil and bake for 35 minutes, or until the noodles have cooked through. Remove from the oven and let cool for at least 15 minutes before cutting and serving. Refrigerate for up to 3 days.

SPINACH

RED BELL PEPPER

YELLOW ONION

CREMINI MUSHROOMS

GARLIC (CLOVES)

PASTA SAUCE

LASAGNA NOODLES

TOFU RICOTTA

note For a gluten-free version, use brown rice lasagna noodles.

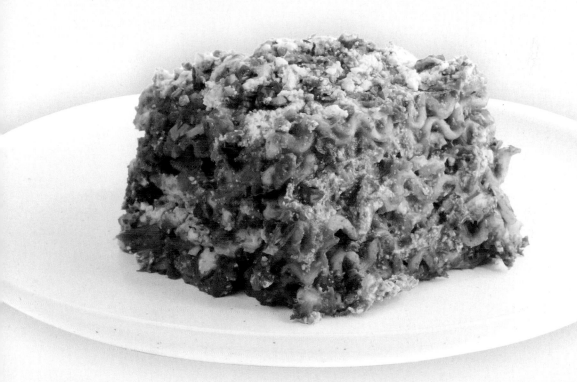

irish stew without the beef or booze

Traditional Irish stew is made by stewing lamb and root vegetables in a thick, gravy-like broth. For my plant-based version, I've opted to use cremini mushrooms, with chunks of carrot, celery, onion, and potato to create a hearty and belly-warming dish. Best served with a big slice of crusty sourdough bread.

MAKES 4 servings (about 1¾ cups per serving) ✦ **FROM START TO FINISH:** 40 minutes

3 celery ribs, chopped

2 carrots, diced

1 medium-size yellow onion, diced

2 garlic cloves, peeled and minced

½ cup all-purpose flour, or as needed

2 tablespoons balsamic vinegar

4½ cups vegetable broth

1 cup cremini mushrooms, diced

4 Yukon Gold potatoes, chopped

¼ cup tomato paste

2 teaspoons dried thyme

1 tablespoon pure maple syrup

2 cups frozen green peas

1. Combine the celery, carrots, onions, and garlic with 2 to 3 tablespoons of water in a large pot. Sauté over medium heat until the onion becomes translucent, 3 to 5 minutes.

2. Sprinkle in ¼ cup of the flour and stir to coat the vegetables. Cook for an additional minute, then add the balsamic vinegar and stir. Finally, add the vegetable broth.

3. Add the mushrooms and potatoes, tomato paste, thyme, and maple syrup (do not add the peas yet). Stir, then simmer, covered, over low heat for 15 to 20 minutes, or until all the vegetables are fork-tender.

4. If the stew needs thickening, combine the remaining ¼ cup of flour with 2 tablespoons of warm water, then pour into the stew. Bring to a quick boil, then lower the heat to help emulsify the flour into the stew.

5. Add the green peas and simmer for an additional 3 minutes, or until they are thawed. Taste and adjust the seasonings as needed. Refrigerate for up to 3 days.

note For a gluten-free version, use a cornstarch slurry (cornstarch and water) to thicken instead.

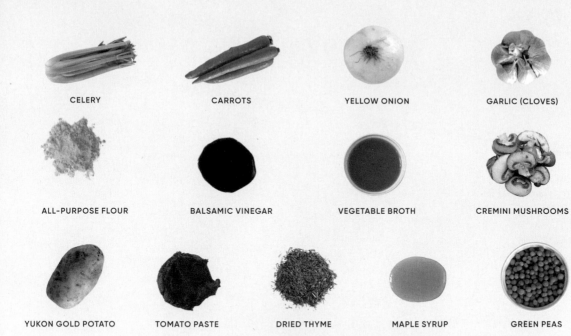

CELERY

CARROTS

YELLOW ONION

GARLIC (CLOVES)

ALL-PURPOSE FLOUR

BALSAMIC VINEGAR

VEGETABLE BROTH

CREMINI MUSHROOMS

YUKON GOLD POTATO

TOMATO PASTE

DRIED THYME

MAPLE SYRUP

GREEN PEAS

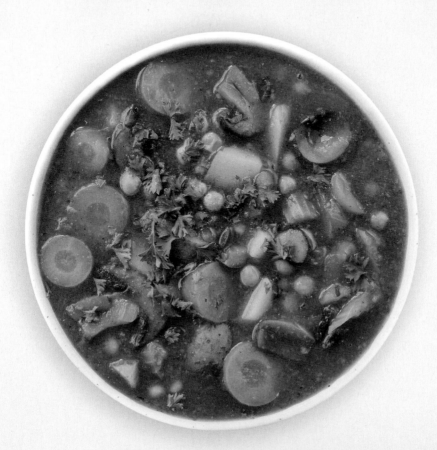

golden shepherd's pie

This hearty pie features a thick medley of vegetables in a savory gravy, topped with creamy golden mashed potatoes. Another perfect recipe around the holidays if you are having guests over for dinner, or for a comforting weeknight meal.

MAKES 6 servings ✦ **FROM START TO FINISH:** 40 minutes

6 Yukon Gold potatoes, peeled and chopped into large chunks

1 teaspoon garlic powder

1 teaspoon onion powder

1 teaspoon salt

2¼ cups vegetable broth

3 carrots, diced

3 celery ribs, chopped

1 medium-size yellow onion, chopped

4 garlic cloves, peeled and minced

2 cups cremini mushrooms, chopped

1 tablespoon tomato paste

3 tablespoons whole wheat flour

2 teaspoons dried thyme

¼ cup balsamic vinegar

1 cup green peas

1. Place the potatoes in a large pot of water, along with the garlic powder, onion powder, and salt. Bring to a boil. Cook for about 15 minutes, or until the potatoes are tender. Drain, then mash, adding ¼ cup of the vegetable broth and additional salt as needed to taste.

2. Combine the carrots, celery, onion, and garlic with 1 tablespoon of the vegetable broth in a large skillet. Cook over medium heat until softened, for 8 to 10 minutes.

3. Add the mushrooms, tomato paste, whole wheat flour, thyme, and balsamic vinegar to the skillet and mix to coat the vegetables. Now, add the remaining vegetable broth, bring to a boil, then lower the heat and stir constantly until thickened.

4. One minute before taking off the heat, add the green peas and stir until they have thawed.

5. Spread the vegetable broth mixture onto the bottom of an 8 x 8-inch baking pan or cast-iron skillet, followed by the mashed potatoes on top. Broil in the middle rack at 500°F for 15 minutes, or until the potatoes start to brown slightly.

note For a gluten-free version, use a cornstarch slurry (cornstarch and water) to thicken instead.

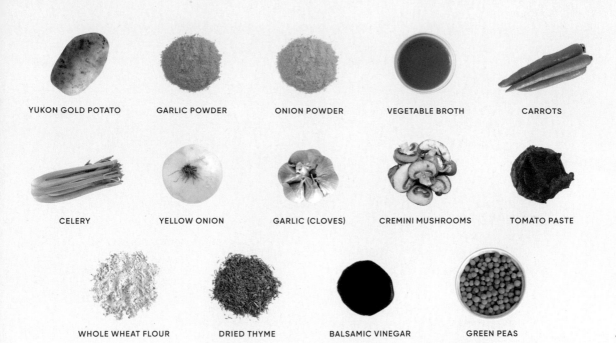

YUKON GOLD POTATO   GARLIC POWDER   ONION POWDER   VEGETABLE BROTH   CARROTS

CELERY   YELLOW ONION   GARLIC (CLOVES)   CREMINI MUSHROOMS   TOMATO PASTE

WHOLE WHEAT FLOUR   DRIED THYME   BALSAMIC VINEGAR   GREEN PEAS

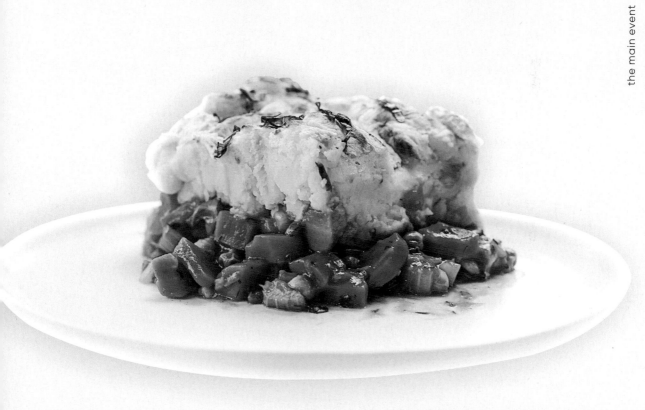

bbq chickpea stuffed
sweet potatoes

This stuffed sweet potato is a fun twist on your standard loaded baked potato. You'll take fluffy sweet potato, top it with crispy barbecue-flavored chickpeas, and finish off with a thick drizzle of a creamy tahini dressing plus fresh-from-the-garden herbs.

MAKES 4 servings ✦ **FROM START TO FINISH:** 50 minutes

4 large sweet potatoes

1 (15-ounce) can chickpeas (about 1½ cups), drained and rinsed

2 teaspoons paprika

1 teaspoon ground cumin

1 teaspoon garlic powder

1 teaspoon chili powder

½ teaspoon salt

¼ cup chopped fresh herbs (I used parsley)

4 servings Classic Tahini Dressing (page 204)

1. Preheat the oven to 400°F. and line a baking sheet with parchment paper.

2. Place the sweet potatoes on one side of the prepared baking sheet, and bake for 45 to 50 minutes, or until soft. Keep in mind that 15 minutes into the sweet potato baking cycle, the seasoned chickpeas need to be placed in the oven to bake as well.

3. Place the chickpeas in a bowl and combine with the paprika, cumin, garlic powder, chili powder, and salt. At the 15-minute point, lay the chickpeas in a single layer next to the sweet potatoes on the prepared baking sheet and bake for the remaining 30 to 35 minutes needed for the sweet potatoes.

4. Once the sweet potatoes and chickpeas are done baking, slice the sweet potatoes in half and mash the insides with a fork. Stuff with the chickpeas and your herbs of choice, and drizzle with the tahini dressing.

SWEET POTATO

CHICKPEAS

PAPRIKA

CUMIN

GARLIC POWDER

CHILI POWDER

PARSLEY

CLASSIC TAHINI
DRESSING

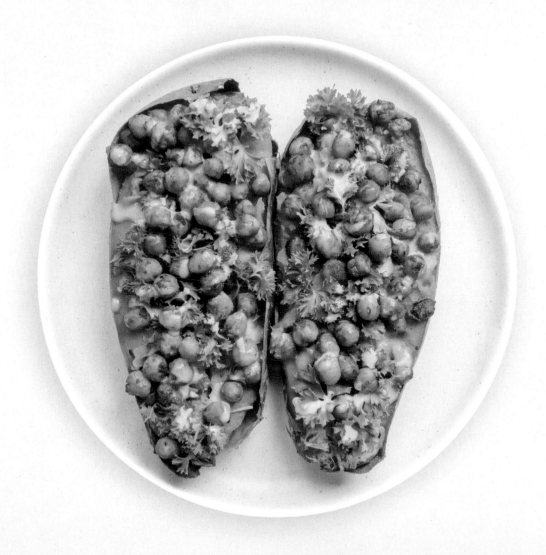

hearty bean & sweet potato chili

In our household, fall is marked by football and a hearty bowl of this bean and sweet potato chili. The addition of sweet potatoes pairs perfectly with the smoky flavor provided by the chili powder and cumin. I use red kidney beans and white navy beans in this recipe, but you can use any of your favorites. This dish also makes for fabulous leftovers, and will keep well in the fridge for up to four days.

MAKES 4 to 6 servings (about 1¾ cups of chili) ✦ **FROM START TO FINISH:** 45 minutes

1 medium-size yellow onion, diced

4 garlic cloves, peeled and minced

2 (28-ounce) cans crushed tomatoes (about 6 cups), with liquid

1 (15-ounce) can red kidney beans (about 1½ cups), drained and rinsed

1 (15-ounce) can white navy beans (about 1½ cups), drained and rinsed

1 cup vegetable broth

1 sweet potato, chopped into 1-inch cubes

2 green bell peppers, seeded and chopped

1 cup cremini mushrooms, minced in a food processor

¼ cup almond butter

3 tablespoons chili powder

2 teaspoons ground cumin

1 teaspoon dried oregano

1 tablespoon salt, or to taste

1. Combine the onion and garlic with 2 tablespoons of water in a large saucepan. Sauté over medium heat until the onion becomes translucent, 2 to 3 minutes.

2. Add all the remaining ingredients to the pot and bring to a boil. Cover and simmer for 35 minutes, or until the sweet potato is fork-tender. Taste and adjust the seasonings as needed. If you would like a thicker consistency, blend a portion of the chili using an immersion blender.

3. Garnish with fresh cilantro and coconut yogurt as desired.

note For a nut-free version, substitute tahini for the almond butter.

YELLOW ONION

GARLIC (CLOVES)

CRUSHED TOMATOES

RED KIDNEY BEANS

WHITE NAVY BEANS

VEGETABLE BROTH

SWEET POTATO

GREEN BELL PEPPER

CREMINI MUSHROOMS

ALMOND BUTTER

CHILI POWDER

CUMIN

OREGANO

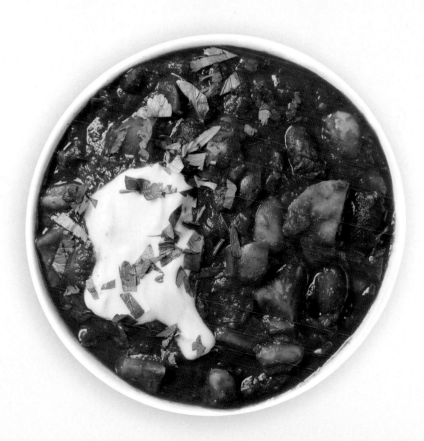

portobello mushroom steaks

As a child, I absolutely despised mushrooms. It's funny how our taste buds change as we get older. I now consider mushrooms one of my favorite foods. They're a staple in vegan cooking, as they naturally have a meat-like texture and will take on the flavor of whichever sauce or marinade you use. This recipe is no exception, in which portobellos develop a divine steak-like flavor after being marinated and baked. These are fabulous served with my Sheet Pan Roasted Vegetables (page 234).

MAKES 4 servings ✦ **FROM START TO FINISH:** 45 minutes

4 large portobello mushrooms

¼ cup red wine vinegar

¼ cup tamari or soy sauce

3 tablespoons pure maple syrup

3 garlic cloves, peeled and minced

1. Preheat the oven to 400°F and line a baking sheet with parchment paper.

2. Wipe the mushrooms with a dry paper towel or clean cloth. Do not wet them or they will become soggy.

3. Whisk together the red wine vinegar, tamari, maple syrup, and garlic in a shallow container large enough to immerse the mushrooms. Add the mushrooms to the container and brush the marinade over their skins. Allow to marinate for 15 minutes.

4. Place the mushrooms, top side down, on the prepared baking sheet and bake for 15 minutes, reserving any leftover marinade.

5. Remove from the oven and turn over the mushrooms, brushing with any remaining marinade at this point. Allow to bake for an additional 15 minutes, or until slightly browned. Serve immediately.

notes

For a more realistic "steak" look, you can take the portobello mushrooms out of the oven five minutes early and place them, top side down, on a barbecue grill, preheated to medium-high, for five minutes.

For a gluten-free version, use wheat-free tamari, not soy sauce.

PORTOBELLO

RED WINE VINEGAR

TAMARI

MAPLE SYRUP

GARLIC (CLOVES)

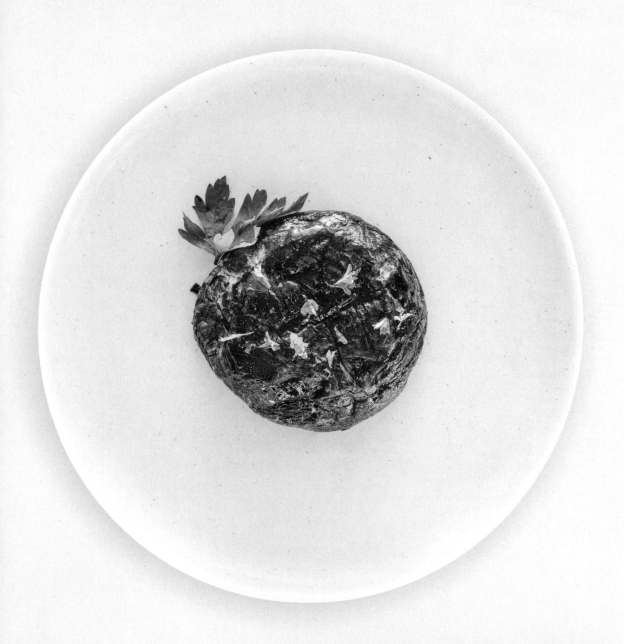

cozy sweet potato peanut stew

If you're looking for a warming recipe that is perfect to enjoy while curled up on the couch under a big fluffy blanket, try this peanut stew! It's another meal that requires just one pot and a list of good-for-you plant-based ingredients, including sweet potato, kale, ginger, and red lentils. This stew is all tied together with a big spoonful of creamy peanut butter, balancing out the fragrant spices.

MAKES 4 to 6 servings (about 1½ cups per serving) ✦ **FROM START TO FINISH:** 50 minutes

1 medium-size yellow onion, diced

3 garlic cloves, peeled and minced

1 red bell pepper, seeded and diced

1 (½-inch-long) piece fresh ginger, peeled and minced

2 medium-size sweet potatoes, diced

1 teaspoon ground cinnamon, Ceylon if possible

1 teaspoon smoked paprika

½ teaspoon ground cumin

½ teaspoon ground turmeric

5 cups vegetable broth

3 tablespoons tomato paste

1 cup dried red lentils

½ cup all-natural peanut butter

2 cups kale, chopped

Salt

Red pepper flakes

1. Combine the onion and garlic with 1 tablespoon of water in a large saucepan. Sauté over medium heat until browned slightly, about 3 minutes.

2. Add the bell pepper, ginger, and sweet potatoes and cook until slightly softened, about 5 minutes.

3. Stir in the cinnamon, smoked paprika, cumin, and turmeric and let the spices cook for 1 minute.

4. Then add the vegetable broth and tomato paste and bring to a boil. Lower the heat to simmer, uncovered, for 20 minutes, or until the sweet potatoes are fork-tender.

5. Stir in the red lentils and peanut butter and simmer until they are cooked, about 10 minutes.

6. Remove from the heat and allow the soup to cool slightly. Transfer half to a countertop blender, or simply use a handheld blender to puree half the stew.

7. Finally, stir in the kale and allow it to wilt. Taste and season with salt and red pepper flakes, as desired.

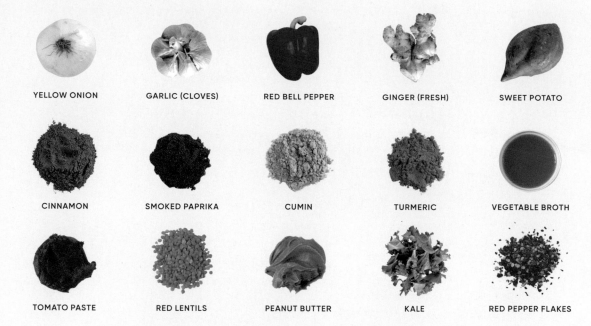

YELLOW ONION **GARLIC (CLOVES)** **RED BELL PEPPER** **GINGER (FRESH)** **SWEET POTATO**

CINNAMON **SMOKED PAPRIKA** **CUMIN** **TURMERIC** **VEGETABLE BROTH**

TOMATO PASTE **RED LENTILS** **PEANUT BUTTER** **KALE** **RED PEPPER FLAKES**

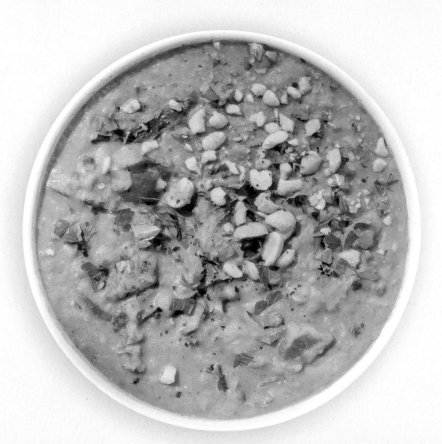

notes

If you don't have vegetable broth, I would suggest water and a vegan bouillon cube for the best flavor.

For a peanut-free version, use tahini instead.

bliss burgers

The consistency of a veggie burger is everything. You don't want it so mushy that it falls apart, but at the same time it's important to avoid an overly tough patty. After several rounds of testing and kitchen fails, I was able to create the quintessential veggie burger that I believe captures the perfect meaty consistency and neutral flavor. Like almost all my recipes, these veggie burgers are also made up of entirely whole food, plant-based ingredients.

MAKES 4 servings ✦ **FROM START TO FINISH:** 30 minutes

¾ cup canned black beans, drained and rinsed, then dried with a paper towel

¾ cup cooked brown rice

½ medium-size yellow onion, chopped

3 tablespoons rolled oats

1 teaspoon garlic powder

1 tablespoon tamari or soy sauce

½ teaspoon chili powder

½ teaspoon smoked paprika

½ teaspoon salt

4 vegan whole wheat burger buns

Your favorite toppings

1. Preheat the oven to 400°F and line a baking sheet with parchment paper.

2. Combine all the ingredients, except for the burger buns and toppings, in a food processor and process until a thick, moldable consistency is achieved.

3. Using your hands, form four or five thin patties, around the thickness of an oatmeal cookie.

4. Bake for 10 minutes, then flip the patties and bake for an additional 10 minutes, or until cooked through.

5. Remove from the oven and allow to cool for 5 minutes before eating. Enjoy in a whole wheat bun with your preferred burger toppings.

note For a gluten-free version, use wheat-free tamari, not soy sauce, and gluten-free buns.

BLACK BEANS

BROWN RICE

YELLOW ONION

ROLLED OATS

GARLIC POWDER

TAMARI

CHILI POWDER

SMOKED PAPRIKA

HAMBURGER BUNS

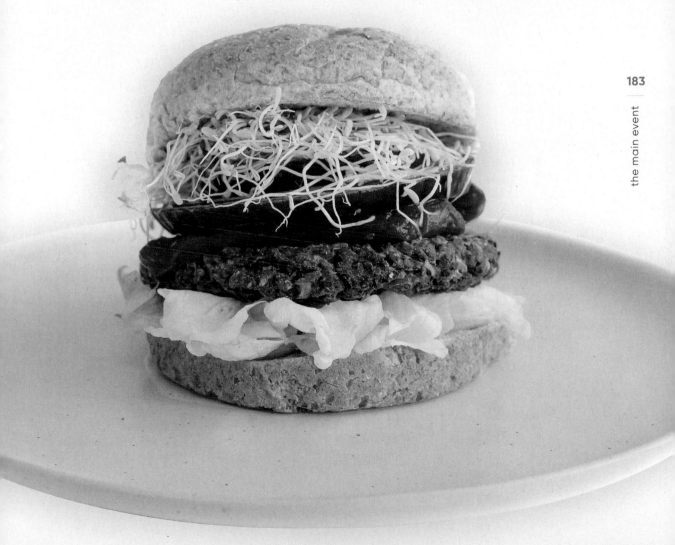

best-ever cauli wings

Instead of a thick flour batter that never really makes the grade, I opted to wrap my cauliflower in edible rice paper as an experiment to emulate a real chicken wing. The result was nothing short of amazing. Rice paper can be a bit challenging to work with, but I promise it will be worth it! You simply soak the rice paper in vegetable broth, then wrap it around the florets. It doesn't have to be a perfect wrapping job, because you're baking them and tossing them in sauce afterward. These cauliflower wings are light, crispy, and insanely delicious, best enjoyed immediately smothered in your favorite wing sauce. I used red hot buffalo sauce for the purpose of this recipe.

MAKES 4 servings (8 wings per serving, depending on your florets)

FROM START TO FINISH: 25 minutes

4 cups vegetable broth

1 medium-size head cauliflower, broken into about 32 florets

16 rice paper wraps

¾ cup red hot sauce

1. Bring the vegetable broth to a boil in a large saucepan over medium heat. Drop in five cauliflower florets at a time, and parboil for 1 minute per batch, removing with a slotted spoon. Repeat until all florets have been parboiled. Allow them to cool for 5 minutes until they can be safely handled.

2. Take the pot off the heat and allow to cool slightly. Slice the rice paper wraps in half with a pair of kitchen scissors, and dip them into the broth for about 10 seconds, or until softened.

3. Wrap an individual rice paper half over each of the cauliflower florets until they are covered completely. Place on a baking sheet and broil at 500°F in the middle rack for 8 minutes, watching and turning about every 2 minutes as they brown.

4. Once lightly crisped, remove from the oven and allow to cool for 10 minutes before tossing in the hot sauce, or your preferred sauce of choice. Enjoy immediately.

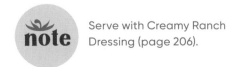

note Serve with Creamy Ranch Dressing (page 206).

VEGETABLE BROTH

CAULIFLOWER

RICE PAPER

HOT SAUCE

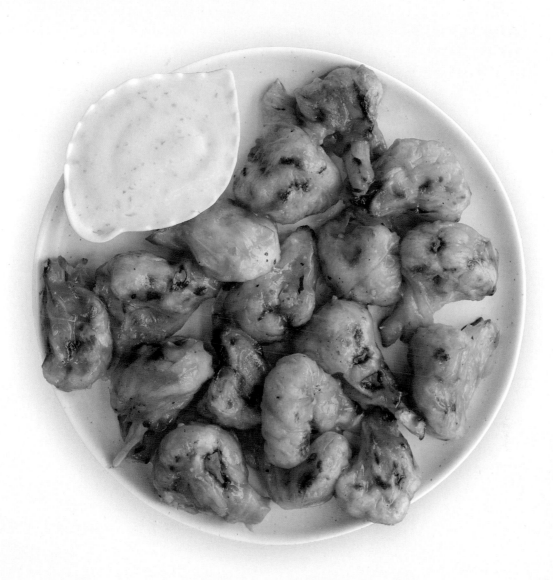

bbq jackfruit pulled pork

If you've never tried jackfruit pulled pork sandwiches, you'll surely do a double take at how much this dish tastes like meat. Despite its being from the fruit family, jackfruit is an amazing meat substitute because of its texture, which is similar to shredded chicken or pork. On its own, it has a bland taste, but will take on the flavor of whatever you cook it in. The key to getting the right texture and flavor is to purchase canned young green jackfruit in water or brine, not syrup, and certainly not the massive fruit you've likely seen. You can find this at most natural food stores or online. I use my Smokin' BBQ Sauce (page 206) for this recipe, but you can use any of your favorite store-bought versions to make life easy.

MAKES 4 servings ✦ **FROM START TO FINISH:** 50 minutes

2 (20-ounce) cans young green jackfruit (about 3 cups), in brine or water, not syrup

1 medium-size yellow onion, diced

4 garlic cloves, minced

1 cup Smokin' BBQ Sauce (page 206)

4 vegan whole wheat burger buns

1. Preheat the oven to 400°F and line a baking sheet with parchment paper.

2. Drain and rinse the jackfruit. Lay the jackfruit on a cutting board and dry it well with a clean cloth or paper towel.

3. Once dry, slice the jackfruit with a knife until it has a shredded consistency.

4. Place the jackfruit in a bowl along with the onion, garlic, and ¾ cup of the barbecue sauce. Mix until well combined.

5. Spread the jackfruit on the prepared baking sheet and bake for 35 minutes.

6. Remove from the oven and brush with the remaining ¼ cup of barbecue sauce. Bake for an additional 10 minutes, or until slightly crisped.

7. Serve in a bun with your desired burger toppings, or as a taco filling.

note For a gluten-free version, serve the jackfruit pulled pork in a gluten-free bun or on top of a salad.

JACKFRUIT

 YELLOW ONION

 GARLIC (CLOVES)

 SMOKIN' BBQ SAUCE

 HAMBURGER BUNS

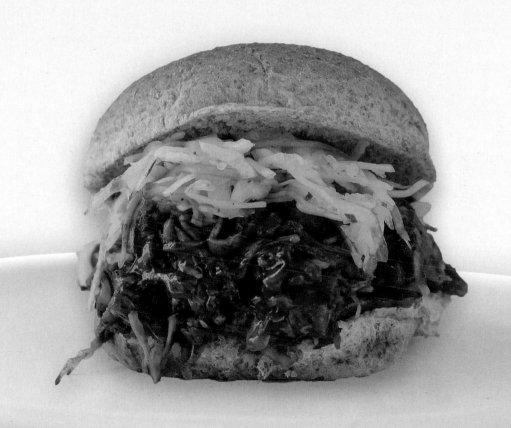

mac 'n' peas

This recipe tastes phenomenal with my Everything Cheeze Sauce (page 212), which is completely nut- and gluten-free (a.k.a. allergy-friendly)! You'll be so shocked to learn you can make a thick, cheddar-yellow sauce using boiled potatoes and carrots. This dish is best served up with green peas or broccoli, both of which will add fiber, nutrients, and protein to your dish!

MAKES 4 servings ✦ **FROM START TO FINISH:** 30 minutes

1 (16-ounce) package whole wheat macaroni pasta

2 Yukon Gold potatoes, peeled and chopped

2 medium-size carrots, chopped

3 tablespoons pickled banana peppers

1 tablespoon garlic powder

1 teaspoon smoked paprika

1 teaspoon freshly squeezed lemon juice

1½ teaspoons salt

3 tablespoons nutritional yeast (optional)

1½ cups frozen peas, thawed

1. Cook the macaroni pasta according to the package directions, until al dente.

2. Meanwhile, place the potatoes and carrots in a large saucepan, fill with water, and bring to a boil. Let boil for 10 to 15 minutes, or until fork-tender. With a slotted spoon, transfer the potatoes and carrots to a countertop blender, along with ½ cup of the cooking liquid.

3. Add the banana peppers, garlic powder, smoked paprika, lemon juice, salt, and nutritional yeast (if using) to the mixture in the blender and combine until velvety smooth. You may need to add 1 to 3 tablespoons of potato water to the blender, as needed, to thin.

4. Taste and adjust the salt and seasonings as needed.

5. Working 1 cup at a time, pour the sauce onto the cooked macaroni and gently stir until fully coated to your desired sauciness. There may be some leftover sauce, which you can use as a chip dip or over roasted vegetables. Stir in the green peas and serve.

note For a gluten-free version, use brown rice macaroni noodles instead.

MACARONI

YUKON GOLD POTATO

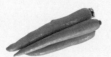

CARROTS

BANANA PEPPERS

GARLIC POWDER

SMOKED PAPRIKA

LEMON (JUICE)

NUTRITIONAL YEAST
(OPTIONAL)

GREEN PEAS

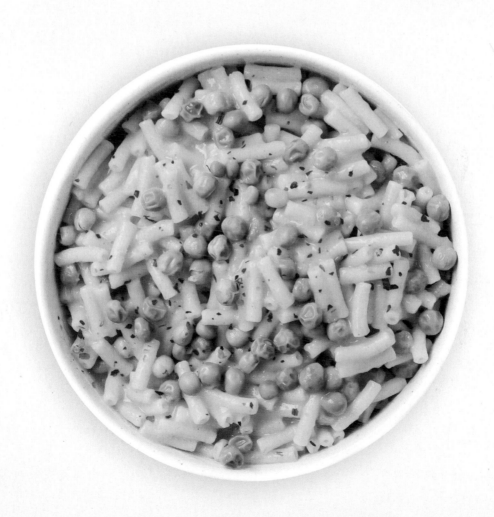

meaty vegan lentil loaf

This hearty and delicious lentil loaf is perfect to serve at any special or holiday dinner, paired with mashed potatoes and green beans. The thick, sliceable texture is achieved by combining lentils, chickpeas, and bread crumbs in a food processor along with sautéed vegetables.

MAKES 6 servings ✦ **FROM START TO FINISH:** 55 minutes

½ medium-size yellow onion, finely chopped

1 red bell pepper, seeded and finely chopped

1 medium-size carrot, peeled and finely chopped

1 cup finely chopped cremini mushrooms

¼ cup ketchup

¼ cup balsamic vinegar

1 (15-ounce) can chickpeas (about 1½ cups), drained and rinsed

1 (15-ounce) can green lentils (about 1½ cups), drained and rinsed

1 cup vegan panko bread crumbs

¼ cup chopped fresh parsley, plus more for garnish

3 tablespoons tamari or soy sauce

1 tablespoon garlic powder

1 tablespoon smoked paprika

1. Preheat the oven to 400°F and line an 8½ x 4½-inch loaf pan with parchment paper.

2. Combine the onion, red bell pepper, carrot, and mushrooms with 1 tablespoon of water in a skillet and cook over medium heat until softened, 6 to 8 minutes.

3. Mix the ketchup and balsamic vinegar in a small bowl. Half of this will be used in the batter, and the other half on top of the loaf.

4. Combine the chickpeas and green lentils in a food processor and process until a chunky paste forms. Transfer to a bowl and mix in the cooked vegetables, panko bread crumbs, parsley, tamari, garlic powder, paprika, and 3 tablespoons of the ketchup mixture.

5. Transfer to the prepared loaf pan and flatten the top of the mixture. Spread on the remaining ketchup-vinegar mixture with the back of a spoon. Bake for 45 minutes, or until firm and cooked through. Remove from the oven and allow to cool for at least 15 minutes before cutting.

 note

For a gluten-free version, simply replace the panko bread crumbs with a gluten-free alternative, and use wheat-free tamari, not soy sauce.

YELLOW ONION

RED BELL PEPPER

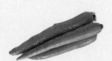

CARROT

CREMINI MUSHROOMS

KETCHUP

BALSAMIC VINEGAR

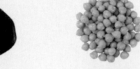

CHICKPEAS

GREEN LENTILS

PANKO BREAD CRUMBS

PARSLEY

TAMARI

GARLIC POWDER

SMOKED PAPRIKA

191

the main event

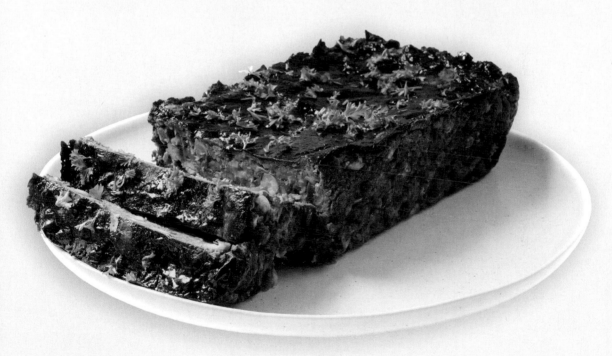

tgif pizza

Friday is pizza night in our home, and bar none, this is my favorite combination for an amazing homemade pizza that will wow both carnivores and vegans alike. To make life easy, I use premade packages of fresh whole wheat pizza dough, which you can find at most mainstream grocery stores or Italian bakeries. Any experience I have had making my own whole wheat dough in the past has ended in disaster with flour and dough everywhere but the countertop, so I can't in good faith recommend it. If you don't love the topping choices listed, feel free to customize this with your favorites!

MAKES 4 servings ✦ **FROM START TO FINISH:** 35 minutes

All-purpose flour, for dusting

1 (16-ounce) package fresh whole wheat pizza dough

1 (15-ounce) can tomato sauce (about 1½ cups)

1 tablespoon Italian seasoning

4 servings Vegan Mozzarella (page 213)

1 cup artichoke hearts, marinated in brine or vinegar, chopped

1 vine-ripened tomato, sliced

1 cup fresh basil

1 cup cremini mushrooms, chopped

1 tablespoon cornmeal

1. Preheat the oven to 425°F.

2. Flour a clean and flat surface, roll out the pizza dough, and transfer to a pizza pan or large, rectangular baking sheet.

3. Top with your desired amount of tomato sauce and then sprinkle with the Italian seasoning.

4. Pour a generous amount of the Vegan Mozzarella sauce directly from the blender onto the pizza, either in blobs to give a mozzarella effect or in streaks across the entire surface.

5. **Next, add the toppings:** the artichoke, sliced tomato, fresh basil, and mushrooms. Finish off by sprinkling cornmeal on the outer edges of the crust.

6. Bake for 17 to 20 minutes, or until crisp and golden brown. Slice into about eight pieces.

note

For a gluten-free version, use a gluten-free pizza crust instead, and gluten-free flour to dust.

PIZZA DOUGH

TOMATO SAUCE

ITALIAN SEASONING

VEGAN MOZZARELLA

ARTICHOKES

VINE-RIPENED TOMATOES

BASIL

CREMINI MUSHROOMS

CORNMEAL

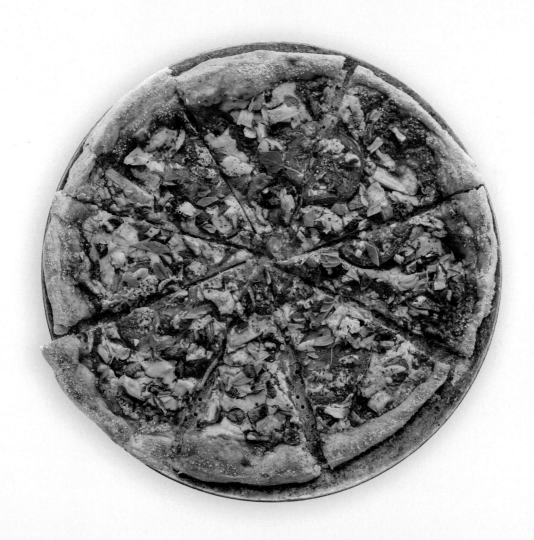

let's get saucy

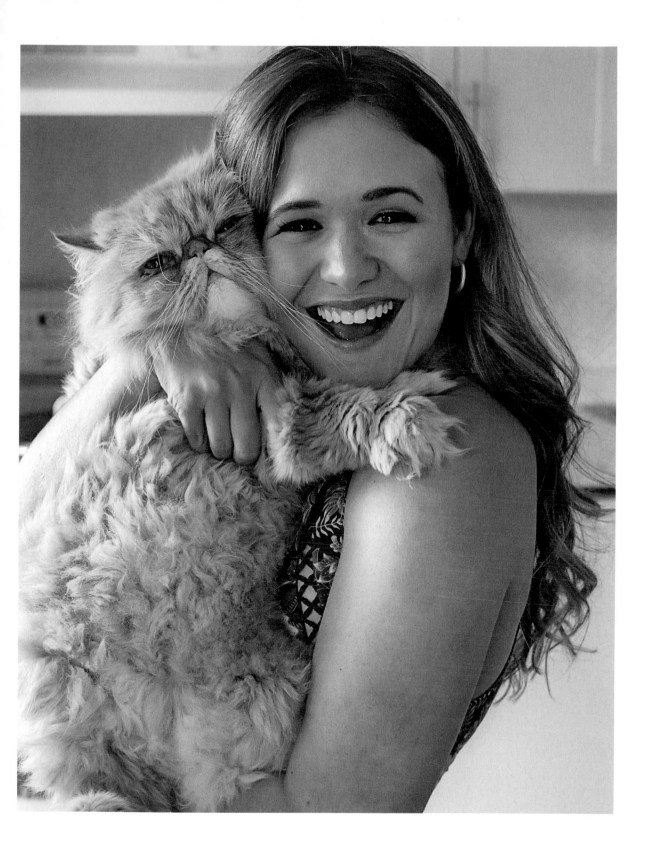

HUMMUS 3 WAYS

For many vegans, hummus is its own food group, slathered on anything from pita bread to pasta. That's why I've included three different delicious ways to prepare hummus to satisfy every taste! Store all of these in a sealed container in the fridge for up to one week.

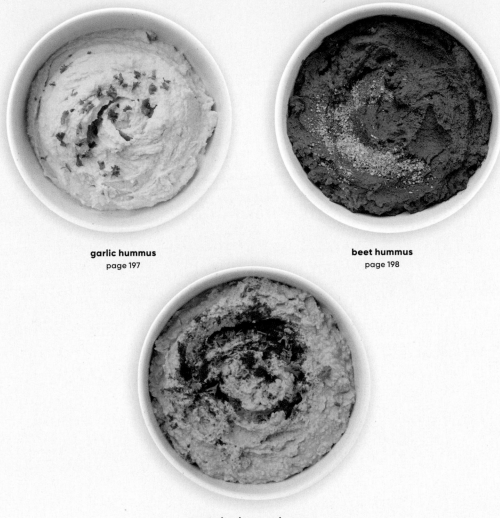

garlic hummus
page 197

beet hummus
page 198

roasted red pepper hummus
page 199

garlic hummus

1 (15-ounce) can chickpeas (about 1½ cups), drained and rinsed

¼ cup tahini

2 garlic cloves, peeled

1 teaspoon freshly squeezed lemon juice

2 tablespoons water, or more as needed

½ teaspoon salt

Fresh parsley, for garnish (optional)

Paprika, for garnish (optional)

Combine all the ingredients, except the garnishes, in a food processor and process until smooth. Garnish with fresh parsley and paprika, as desired. Store in a sealed container in the fridge for up to 1 week.

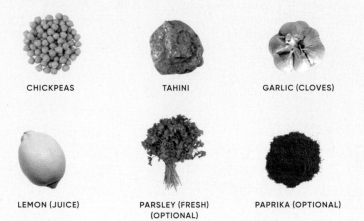

CHICKPEAS

TAHINI

GARLIC (CLOVES)

LEMON (JUICE)

PARSLEY (FRESH) (OPTIONAL)

PAPRIKA (OPTIONAL)

197

let's get saucy

beet hummus

MAKES 6 servings (about ⅓ cup per serving) ✦ **FROM START TO FINISH:** 1 hour 45 minutes

1 medium-size beet

1 (15-ounce) can chickpeas (about 1½ cups), drained and rinsed

¼ cup tahini

2 garlic cloves, peeled

2 teaspoons freshly squeezed lemon juice

1 tablespoon water

½ teaspoon salt

Fresh parsley, for garnish (optional)

Ground flaxseeds, for garnish (optional)

1. Preheat the oven to 400°F and wrap the beet in foil. Roast for 1½ hours, or until the beet is soft and tender.

2. Once the beet is roasted, remove it from the oven and allow it to cool. Once cool, peel off the skin and cut the beet into chunks.

3. Place the beet chunks in a food processor and process until ground. Now, add the rest of the ingredients, except the garnishes, to the food processor and process until a smooth hummus is formed.

4. Garnish with parsley or ground flaxseeds, as desired. Store in the fridge in a sealed container for up to 1 week.

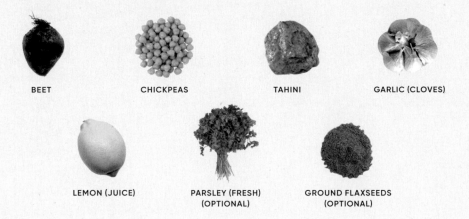

BEET   CHICKPEAS   TAHINI   GARLIC (CLOVES)

LEMON (JUICE)   PARSLEY (FRESH)   GROUND FLAXSEEDS
                  (OPTIONAL)   (OPTIONAL)

roasted red pepper hummus

MAKES 6 servings (about ⅓ cup per serving) ✦ **FROM START TO FINISH:** 10 minutes

1 (15-ounce) can chickpeas (about 1½ cups), drained and rinsed

⅔ cup jarred roasted red peppers, drained

2 tablespoons tahini

2 cloves garlic, peeled

2 tablespoons freshly squeezed lemon juice

½ teaspoon salt

3 tablespoons water

Fresh parsley, for garnish (optional)

Paprika, for garnish (optional)

Combine all the ingredients, except the garnishes, in a food processor until smooth. Garnish with fresh parsley and paprika, as desired. Store in a sealed container in the fridge for up to 1 week.

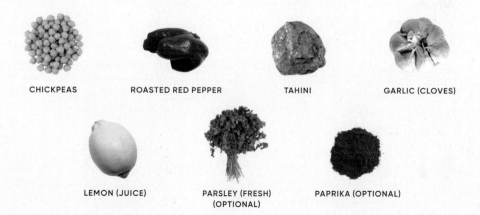

CHICKPEAS   ROASTED RED PEPPER   TAHINI   GARLIC (CLOVES)

LEMON (JUICE)   PARSLEY (FRESH) (OPTIONAL)   PAPRIKA (OPTIONAL)

salad dressings & sauces

Mastering a whole food, plant-based, oil-free lifestyle can be extremely challenging if you don't have some go-to salad dressings and sauces on hand. And contrary to popular belief, oil is not a required ingredient for salad dressings! This section has eight different salad dressings and sauces, from an everyday balsamic to a smokin' BBQ sauce. All of these should last safely in the fridge in sealed containers for about one week.

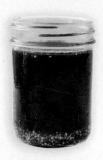

go-to balsamic
page 202

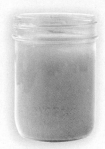

apple cider vinaigrette
page 202

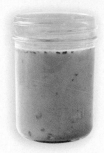

spicy peanut dressing
page 203

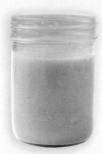

classic tahini dressing
page 204

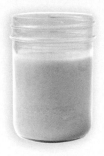

turmeric tahini dressing
page 204

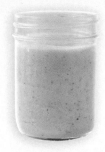

cilantro lime dressing
page 205

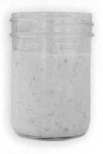

creamy ranch dressing
page 206

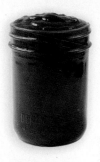

smokin' bbq sauce
page 206

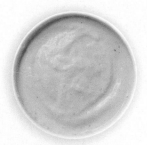

cashew mayo
page 207

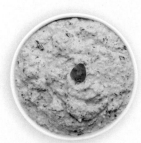

spinach basil pesto
page 208

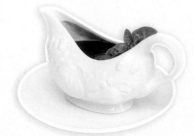

easy vegan gravy
page 209

go-to balsamic

Best all-purpose salad dressing for dishes like the Balsamic Pasta Salad (page 120), Superloaded Veggie Wrap (page 104), or any side salad rich in leafy greens, such as arugula, kale, or spinach.

MAKES 4 to 6 servings (about 1½ tablespoons per serving) ✦ **FROM START TO FINISH:** 1 minute

6 tablespoons balsamic vinegar

1 tablespoon Dijon mustard

1½ teaspoons pure maple syrup

1½ teaspoons dried basil

1½ teaspoons garlic powder

1½ teaspoons sea salt

Whisk together all the ingredients in a small bowl or jar until completely combined.

BALSAMIC VINEGAR   DIJON MUSTARD   MAPLE SYRUP   DRIED BASIL   GARLIC POWDER

apple cider vinaigrette

Best served with the Quinoa Cranberry Harvest Salad (page 128) or as a light, all-purpose salad dressing with arugula or spinach.

MAKES 6 servings (about 2½ tablespoons per serving) ✦ **FROM START TO FINISH:** 1 minute

½ cup apple juice

2 tablespoons cider vinegar

2 teaspoons Dijon mustard

Pinch of sea salt

Whisk together all the ingredients in a small bowl or jar until completely combined.

APPLE JUICE   CIDER VINEGAR   DIJON MUSTARD

spicy peanut dressing

Best served with the Crunchy Peanut Shredded Salad (page 122), as a peanut sauce for stir-fries, or drizzled over nourishing bowls.

MAKES 4 servings (about 3 tablespoons per serving) ✦ **FROM START TO FINISH:** 1 minute

¼ cup smooth, all-natural peanut butter

3 tablespoons tamari or soy sauce

1 tablespoon pure maple syrup

1 tablespoon cider vinegar

Juice of ½ lime

¼ teaspoon red pepper flakes

3 tablespoons warm water, or more to thin

Whisk together all the ingredients in a small bowl or jar until completely combined.

PEANUT BUTTER   TAMARI   MAPLE SYRUP   CIDER VINEGAR   LIME (JUICE)   RED PEPPER FLAKES

let's get saucy

notes

For a peanut-free version, use a soy-based peanut butter alternative or tahini instead of peanut butter.

For a gluten-free version, use wheat-free tamari, not soy sauce.

classic tahini dressing

Best served with the BBQ Chickpea Stuffed Sweet Potatoes (page 174) or as an all-purpose salad dressing for a heartier salad with quinoa or rice, or drizzled over roasted vegetables.

MAKES 4 servings (about 2 tablespoons per serving) ✦ **FROM START TO FINISH:** 1 minute

⅓ cup tahini

2 tablespoons freshly squeezed lemon juice

1 tablespoon pure maple syrup

¼ cup water, or more to thin

Whisk together all the ingredients in a small bowl or jar until completely combined.

TAHINI

LEMON (JUICE)

MAPLE SYRUP

turmeric tahini dressing

Best served with the Build-a-Bowl (page 114) or as an all-purpose salad dressing or drizzled over a nourishing bowl or roasted vegetables.

MAKES 4 servings (about 2 tablespoons per serving) ✦ **FROM START TO FINISH:** 1 minute

⅓ cup tahini

1 teaspoon pure maple syrup

½ teaspoon ground turmeric

½ teaspoon of salt

Pinch of freshly ground black pepper

¼ cup water, or more to thin

Whisk together all the ingredients in a small bowl or jar until completely combined.

TAHINI

MAPLE SYRUP

TURMERIC

cilantro lime dressing

Best served with the Roasted Corn, Bell Pepper & Cilantro Salad (page 130), or as an all-purpose salad dressing that pairs well with avocado, red onion, and tomato.

MAKES 3 to 4 servings (about 1½ tablespoons per serving) ✦ **FROM START TO FINISH:** 5 minutes

1 ripe avocado, peeled and pitted
⅓ cup unsweetened almond milk
Juice of ½ lime

½ cup fresh cilantro
½ teaspoon sea salt

Combine all the ingredients in a blender and blend until completely smooth.

AVOCADO

ALMOND MILK

LIME (JUICE)

CILANTRO

note For a nut-free version, use soy milk instead.

let's get saucy

creamy ranch dressing

Best served with the Cool Ranch Kale Salad (page 124), in the Buffalo Chick'n Wrap (page 110), or as a vegetable dip.

MAKES 4 to 6 servings (about 3½ tablespoons per serving) ✦ **FROM START TO FINISH:** 5 minutes

10 ounces silken tofu

1 tablespoon cider vinegar

¾ tablespoon warm water

¾ teaspoon garlic powder, or 2 garlic cloves, minced

½ teaspoon sea salt

1 teaspoon dried parsley

Combine all the ingredients in a blender and blend until completely smooth.

SILKEN TOFU   CIDER VINEGAR   GARLIC POWDER   DRIED PARSLEY

let's get saucy

smokin' bbq sauce

Best served with the BBQ Jackfruit Pulled Pork (page 186), with vegan tacos, or in a chili.

MAKES 4 to 6 servings (about 3½ tablespoons per serving) ✦ **FROM START TO FINISH:** 1 minute

1 cup organic low-sugar ketchup

¼ cup cider vinegar

2 tablespoons pure maple syrup

1½ tablespoons soy sauce

1½ tablespoons smoked paprika

1 tablespoon garlic powder

Whisk together all the ingredients in a small bowl or jar until completely combined.

KETCHUP   CIDER VINEGAR   MAPLE SYRUP   SOY SAUCE   SMOKED PAPRIKA   GARLIC POWDER

cashew mayo

Best served with sandwiches, wraps, potato salad, and on corn on the cob.

MAKES 12 servings (about 2 tablespoons per serving) ✦ **FROM START TO FINISH:** 5 minutes

1 cup raw cashews, soaked in water overnight or boiled for 15 minutes

¼ cup water, or more as needed

1 tablespoon cider vinegar

1 teaspoon garlic powder

1 teaspoon Dijon mustard

¾ teaspoon sea salt

Combine all the ingredients in a food processor or high-speed blender and process until smooth, adding more water as needed.

CASHEWS

CIDER VINEGAR

GARLIC POWDER

DIJON MUSTARD

note For a nut-free version, substitute a 12-ounce package of silken tofu. Store in the fridge for up to 1 week.

let's get saucy

spinach basil pesto

Best served with our Presto Pesto Penne (page 134), as a sauce base on pizza or flatbread, as a veggie dip, or on roasted veggies.

MAKES 4 to 6 servings (4 to 6 tablespoons per serving)   **FROM START TO FINISH:** 5 minutes

2 cups fresh basil

2 cups spinach

3 garlic cloves, peeled

1 vine-ripened tomato

2 tablespoons freshly squeezed lemon juice

1 teaspoon salt

¾ cup pine nuts or cashews

Combine all the ingredients, except for the pine nuts, in a food processor or high-speed blender and process until smooth. Add the pine nuts and blend until a smooth pesto paste is formed.

let's get saucy

BASIL (FRESH)   SPINACH   GARLIC (CLOVES)   VINE-RIPENED TOMATOES   LEMON (JUICE)   PINE NUTS

note For a nut-free version, try soaked sunflower seeds or white beans instead.

easy vegan gravy

Best served with the Meaty Vegan Lentil Loaf (page 190) and Golden Mashed Potatoes (page 222).

If you have ten minutes, you can whip together this amazing gravy! By now, you know I like to keep things simple, which is why this recipe requires just six ingredients and one pot. You can add sautéed mushrooms if you're feeling fancy.

MAKES 6 servings (about 3 tablespoons per serving)   **FROM START TO FINISH:** 10 minutes

1 cup vegetable broth

2 tablespoons tamari or soy sauce

1 teaspoon garlic powder

½ teaspoon dried parsley

¼ teaspoon dried thyme

**1 tablespoon cornstarch or arrowroot +
1 tablespoon warm water**

1. Combine all the ingredients, except the cornstarch, in a small saucepan. Bring to a boil, then simmer over medium heat for 2 minutes.

2. Combine the cornstarch and the warm water in a small bowl and mix until a slurry is achieved, then pour that into the gravy mixture. Whisk vigorously and bring the mixture back to a boil to thicken. Add more slurry, if needed.

VEGETABLE
BROTH   TAMARI   GARLIC
POWDER   DRIED PARSLEY   DRIED THYME   CORNSTARCH

note For a gluten-free version, use wheat-free tamari, not soy sauce.

vegan cheeze sauces

Cheese is definitely one of the most challenging things to part with when you first pursue a plant-based lifestyle. Even more challenging is the fact that most store-bought vegan cheeses seem to be oil based, and leave you with that same heavy gut feeling as dairy cheeses. That's why I've provided five different "cheeze"-style sauces for every occasion. All of these should last safely in the fridge in sealed containers for four to five days.

For all recipes, for a nut-free version, use soaked sunflower seeds or white beans in place of cashews, and use water or soy milk to blend.

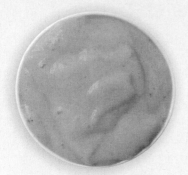

everything cheeze sauce
page 212

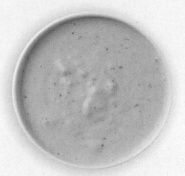

vegan mozzarella
page 213

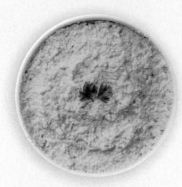

herb & garlic cream cheeze
page 214

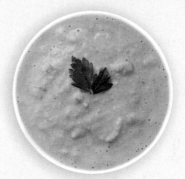

vegan queso
page 214

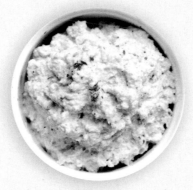

tofu ricotta
page 215

everything cheeze sauce

Best served with the Mac 'n' Peas (page 188), Garlic Asparagus with Cheeze Sauce (page 228), or as an allergy-friendly chip dip.

MAKES 4 to 6 servings (about ¾ cup per serving) ✦ **FROM START TO FINISH:** 25 minutes

2 Yukon Gold potatoes, peeled and chopped

2 medium-size carrots, chopped

3 tablespoons pickled banana peppers

1 tablespoon garlic powder

1 teaspoon smoked paprika

1 teaspoon freshly squeezed lemon juice

1½ teaspoons sea salt

3 tablespoons nutritional yeast (optional)

3 tablespoons unsweetened rice milk (optional), or any neutral plant-based milk

1. Place the potatoes and carrots in a large saucepan or soup pot with enough water to cover by an inch and bring to a boil. Boil for 10 to 15 minutes, or until fork-tender. With a slotted spoon, transfer the potatoes and carrots to a countertop blender, along with ½ cup of the cooking liquid. Reserve the remaining cooking liquid, just in case, for thinning.

2. Next, add the banana peppers, garlic powder, smoked paprika, lemon juice, sea salt, and nutritional yeast (if using) to the blender and blend until velvety smooth. You may need to add 1 to 3 tablespoons of the reserved cooking liquid or rice milk to the blender to thin. Taste and adjust the salt and seasonings as needed. Store in the fridge for up to 3 days.

YUKON GOLD POTATO

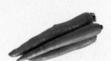

CARROTS

BANANA PEPPERS

GARLIC POWDER

SMOKED PAPRIKA

LEMON (JUICE)

NUTRITIONAL YEAST (OPTIONAL)

RICE MILK (OPTIONAL)

note This recipe is nut-, soy-, and gluten-free.

vegan mozzarella

Best served on the TGIF Pizza (page 192), in a baked pasta dish, or as cheese curds over a poutine, for my Canadian friends.

MAKES 6 to 8 servings (about 3 tablespoons per serving) ✦ **FROM START TO FINISH:** 5 minutes

1 cup raw cashews, soaked in water overnight or boiled for 15 minutes

½ cup unsweetened coconut yogurt

1 teaspoon cider vinegar

1 teaspoon cornstarch or arrowroot powder

½ teaspoon garlic powder, or 1 garlic clove, minced

1 teaspoon sea salt

Unsweetened almond milk (optional)

1. Combine all the ingredients in a blender and blend until smooth. Add 1 to 4 tablespoons of water or unsweetened almond milk as needed to blend.

2. If you want to make cheese curds, simply place the sauce in a pot and stir over medium heat until the cheese thickens, about 5 minutes.

3. Place in the fridge and spoon out curds of the mozzarella to enjoy. Store in the fridge for up to 3 days.

CASHEWS

COCONUT YOGURT

CIDER VINEGAR

CORNSTARCH

GARLIC POWDER

ALMOND MILK (OPTIONAL)

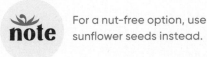

note For a nut-free option, use sunflower seeds instead.

herb & garlic cream cheeze

Best served with a bagel or English muffin, or baked in pasta dishes.

MAKES 6 servings (about 2½ tablespoons per serving) ✦ **FROM START TO FINISH:** 5 minutes

1 cup raw cashews, soaked in water overnight or boiled for 15 minutes

1 teaspoon freshly squeezed lemon juice

1 teaspoon cider vinegar

¼ teaspoon sea salt

2 garlic cloves, peeled

½ teaspoon dried basil

¼ teaspoon dried dill

Combine all the ingredients in a food processor or high-speed blender and process until smooth. Store in the fridge for up to 1 week.

CASHEWS LEMON (JUICE) CIDER VINEGAR GARLIC (CLOVES) DRIED BASIL DRIED DILL

vegan queso

Best served with the Beaming Burrito Bowl (page 116), the Sheet Pan Fajitas (page 144), or as a delicious chip dip.

MAKES 4 to 6 servings (about ¼ cup per serving) ✦ **FROM START TO FINISH:** 5 minutes

½ cup raw cashews, soaked in water overnight or boiled for 15 minutes

½ cup chunky salsa, such as Classic Homemade Salsa (page 219)

1 red bell pepper, seeded and chopped

½ teaspoon ground turmeric

Combine all the ingredients in a blender and blend until smooth. Store in the fridge for up to 4 days.

CASHEWS SALSA RED BELL PEPPER TURMERIC

tofu ricotta

Best served with our "Can't Believe It's Vegan" Lasagna (page 168), over any pasta dish, or spread on toast.

MAKES 4 to 6 servings (about ¼ cup per serving) ✦ **FROM START TO FINISH:** 5 minutes

1 (16-ounce) package extra-firm tofu

3 tablespoons freshly squeezed lemon juice

½ teaspoon salt

1 teaspoon dried basil

1 tablespoon brown rice miso paste, tamari, or soy sauce

1 garlic clove, peeled

1 teaspoon cider vinegar

Combine all the ingredients in a food processor and process until smooth. Store in the fridge for up to 4 days.

| EXTRA-FIRM TOFU | LEMON (JUICE) | DRIED BASIL | MISO PASTE | GARLIC (CLOVE) | CIDER VINEGAR |

notes

You can customize this recipe endlessly by adding your favorite herbs, such as dill, garlic powder, and more.

For a gluten-free version, use wheat-free tamari, not soy sauce.

salsas

Whether you like to use them as a dip or add them to salads, sandwiches, or wraps, salsas are a staple in plant-based cooking. They're an amazing, easy, and light way to add big flavor and nutrients. Of course I couldn't just share one recipe, so here are three of my favorites as well as guacamole as an extra!

To peel tomatoes, you want to blanch them. Slice an X into the bottom of each tomato. With a slotted spoon, place each tomato in boiling water for a few seconds, then into an ice bath. The skins will peel right off.

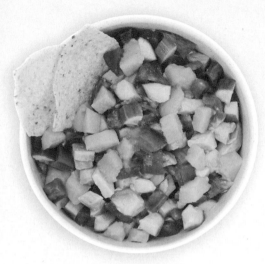

mango salsa
page 218

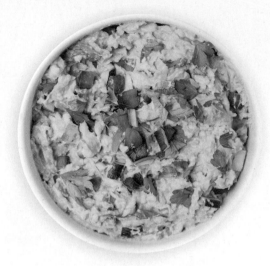

guacamole
page 218

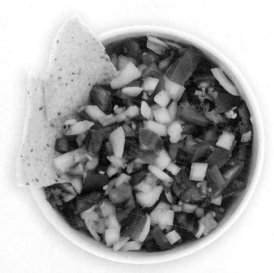

pico de gallo
page 219

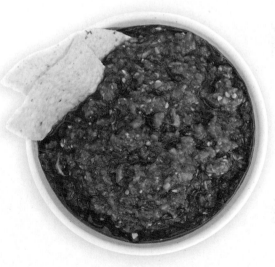

classic homemade salsa
page 219

217

let's get saucy

mango salsa

MAKES 6 servings (about ½ cup salsa per serving) ✦ **FROM START TO FINISH:** 5 minutes

1 mango, peeled, pitted, and diced

2 avocados, pitted, peeled, and diced

2 Roma tomatoes, diced

1 cucumber, diced

Juice of 1 lime

1 garlic clove, peeled and minced

Combine all the ingredients in a bowl and gently toss until mixed. Best paired with crispy nacho chips or on top of tacos. Store in the fridge for up to 2 days.

MANGO

AVOCADO

ROMA TOMATO

CUCUMBER

LIME (JUICE)

GARLIC (CLOVE)

guacamole

MAKES 6 servings (about ½ cup per serving) ✦ **FROM START TO FINISH:** 5 minutes

4 avocados, peeled and pitted

1 garlic clove, peeled and minced

¼ red onion, diced

Juice of 1 lime

1 tomato, diced

¼ teaspoon sea salt

Place the avocado flesh in a bowl and mash with a fork until your desired texture is reached. Add the remaining ingredients and gently stir until combined. Best served with crispy nacho chips or in a burrito. Enjoy immediately.

AVOCADO

GARLIC (CLOVE)

RED ONION

LIME (JUICE)

TOMATO

pico de gallo

5 roma tomatoes, diced

¼ medium-size yellow onion, diced

¼ cup fresh cilantro

Juice of 1 lime

2 garlic cloves, peeled and minced

½ jalapeño pepper, diced

Combine all the ingredients in a bowl and gently stir until well mixed. Best enjoyed on top of a salad or with vegan crackers or nacho chips. Store in the fridge for up to 3 days.

ROMA TOMATO · YELLOW ONION · CILANTRO · LIME (JUICE) · GARLIC (CLOVES) · JALAPEÑO

classic homemade salsa

MAKES 8 to 10 servings (about ½ cup per serving) ✦ **FROM START TO FINISH:** 45 minutes

10 Roma tomatoes, peeled and chopped

1 medium-size yellow onion, chopped

4 garlic cloves, peeled and chopped

¼ cup fresh cilantro, chopped

1 teaspoon cider vinegar

4 jalapeño peppers, seeded and chopped

Pinch of salt

1. Combine all the ingredients, except the salt, in a large pot and simmer for 30 minutes, or until your desired consistency is reached.

2. Season with salt to taste. Allow to cool and transfer to jars. Best served with nacho chips or vegan crackers, or on top of a nourishing bowl. Keeps in the refrigerator for up to a week.

ROMA TOMATO · YELLOW ONION · GARLIC (CLOVES) · CILANTRO · CIDER VINEGAR · JALAPEÑO

simple
sides

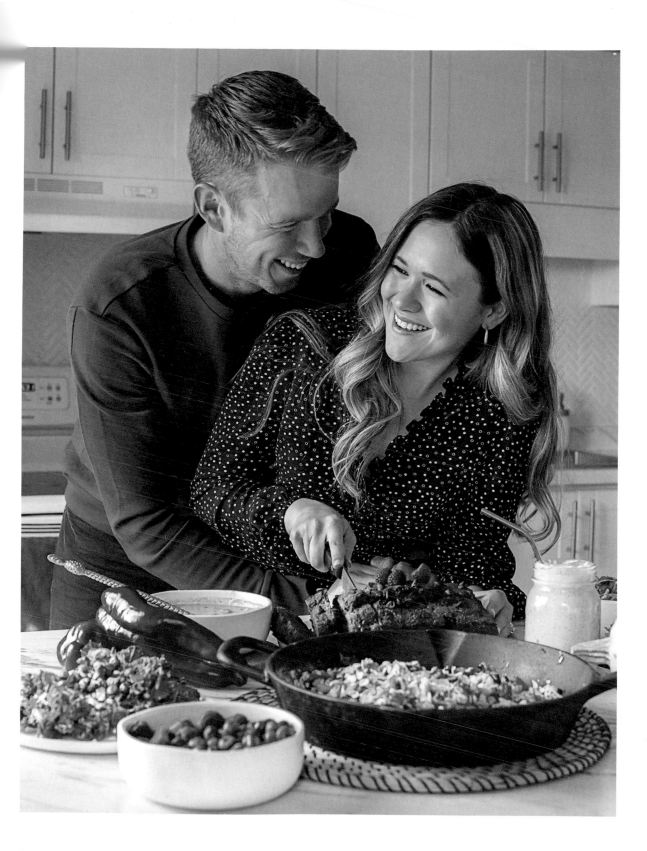

golden mashed potatoes

Move over, butter- and milk-filled mashed potatoes. These need just a few simple ingredients to achieve velvety, fluffy potato goodness, perfect as both a holiday and everyday side dish.

MAKES 6 servings ✦ **FROM START TO FINISH:** 20 minutes

6 Yukon Gold potatoes, peeled

1 teaspoon garlic powder

1 teaspoon onion powder

1 teaspoon salt

¼ cup vegetable broth

1. Place the potatoes in a large pot of water, along with the garlic powder, onion powder, and salt. Bring to a boil.

2. Cook for about 15 minutes, or until the potatoes are tender.

3. Drain, then mash, adding the vegetable broth and additional salt as needed to taste.

YUKON GOLD POTATO

GARLIC POWDER

ONION POWDER

VEGETABLE BROTH

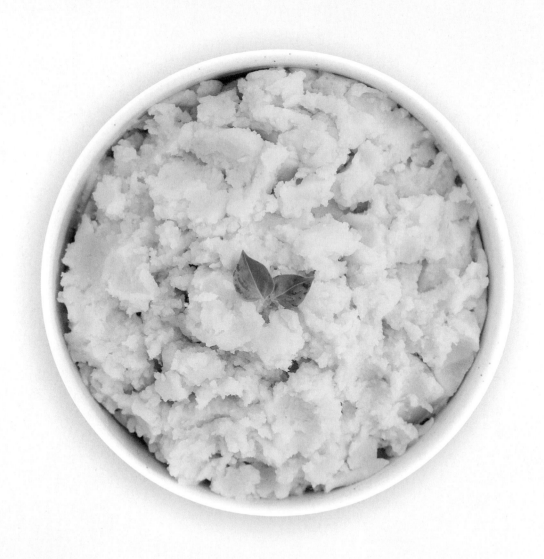

crispy dill french fries

French fries have gotten a bit of a bad rep over the years, and it's because most are deep-fried in oil. As a result, typical fries are pretty heavy. These fries are the opposite, and I promise you won't miss the oil one bit! They're crispy and salty—and the dill adds a delicious twist.

MAKES 4 servings   ✦   **FROM START TO FINISH:** 45 minutes

4 medium-size Yukon Gold potatoes, unpeeled, sliced into wedges

1 tablespoon chopped fresh dill

1 tablespoon garlic powder

1 tablespoon salt

1. Preheat the oven to 375°F and line a baking sheet with parchment paper.

2. Combine the sliced potatoes with the dill, garlic powder, and salt in a bowl and toss until coated.

3. Pour the potato slices onto the baking sheet and roast for 35 minutes, or until crispy.

YUKON GOLD POTATO

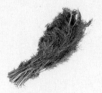

FRESH DILL

GARLIC POWDER

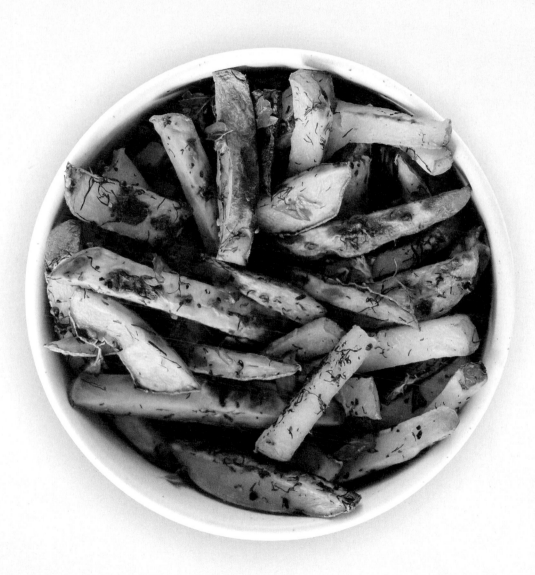

quick pickled red onions

I have a bit of an obsession with these pickled red onions. They take five minutes to whip together, and are amazing on tacos, in wraps, or on top of a salad. Once you learn how to make these, you'll want a jar in the fridge every week. You'll want to use a 16-ounce mason jar or another jar with a sealable lid.

MAKES 6 servings ✦ **FROM START TO FINISH:** 30 minutes

1 cup warm water

1 cup cider vinegar

1 tablespoon coconut sugar

1 teaspoon sea salt

1 red onion, sliced

1. Combine the warm water, cider vinegar, coconut sugar, and sea salt in a bowl to create a brine.

2. Place the red onion slices in a clean jar and pour the brine over the onion. Screw on the lid and place in a warm spot on your counter for 30 minutes.

3. Enjoy immediately, or store in your fridge for up to 1 week.

CIDER VINEGAR

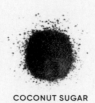

COCONUT SUGAR

RED ONION

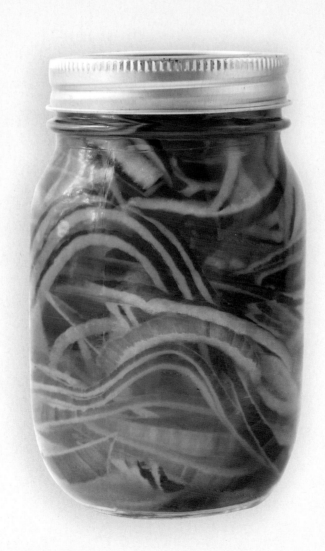

garlic asparagus
with cheeze sauce

As a kid, the only way I would eat asparagus was if it was smothered in Cheez Whiz. Oh, how times have changed. This recipe is inspired by that childhood classic, except way healthier (and tastier too)! This dish is best served in the summertime, with a Bliss Burger (page 182) or BBQ Jackfruit Pulled Pork sandwiches (page 186).

MAKES 4 servings ✦ **FROM START TO FINISH:** 25 minutes

1 bunch thin asparagus, trimmed

1 tablespoon garlic powder

1 teaspoon freshly squeezed lemon juice

½ teaspoon sea salt

¼ cup Everything Cheeze Sauce (page 212)

Fresh parsley, for garnish (optional)

1. Preheat the oven to 400°F and line a baking sheet with parchment paper.

2. Spread the asparagus on the baking sheet and sprinkle with the garlic powder, lemon juice, and sea salt.

3. Bake until tender, 12 to 15 minutes.

4. Pour the cheeze sauce over the asparagus and garnish with fresh parsley, if desired.

ASPARAGUS

GARLIC POWDER

LEMON (JUICE)

**EVERYTHING CHEEZE
SAUCE**

**PARSLEY (FRESH)
(OPTIONAL)**

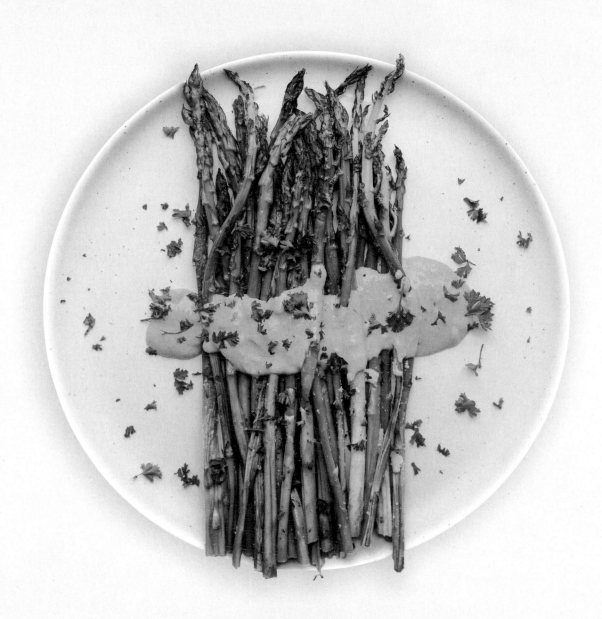

curried bok choy

Did you know bok choy is actually in the cabbage family? It's considered a type of Chinese cabbage, and it's a great vegetable for sautéing because the leaves hold up relatively well. This amazing baby bok choy dish simmered in a curried coconut milk takes just fifteen minutes from start to finish. Excellent served with rice, or to complement a meaty main, such as our Meaty Vegan Lentil Loaf (page 190).

MAKES 4 servings ✦ **FROM START TO FINISH:** 15 minutes

1 pound baby bok choy, cleaned thoroughly, stems trimmed

3 garlic cloves, peeled and minced

2 teaspoons curry powder

2 teaspoons pure maple syrup

½ teaspoon sea salt

½ cup light coconut milk

1. Combine the bok choy, garlic, curry powder, maple syrup, and sea salt in a large skillet with a lid (you will use it later). Sauté over medium heat for 3 to 5 minutes, adding 1 to 2 tablespoons of water, if needed.

2. Add the coconut milk and stir to combine. Lower the heat and cover the pan. Steam the bok choy for 2 to 3 minutes, or until tender.

3. Taste and adjust the flavoring as needed.

BOK CHOY

GARLIC (CLOVES)

CURRY POWDER

MAPLE SYRUP

COCONUT MILK

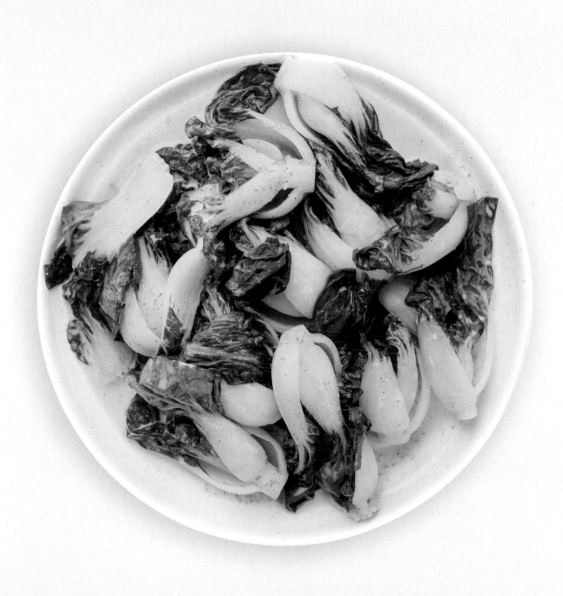

roasted baby potatoes & green beans

Deliciously seasoned with the flavors of garlic and lemon, these potatoes and green beans are the perfect accompaniment to any of my hearty mains, such as the Portobello Mushroom Steaks (page 178), Meaty Vegan Lentil Loaf (page 190), and Bliss Burgers (page 182).

MAKES 4 to 6 servings ✦ **FROM START TO FINISH:** 35 minutes

1½ pounds mini red potatoes, sliced in half

1 red bell pepper, seeded and chopped

1 medium-size yellow onion, chopped

2 cups green beans

¼ cup vegetable broth

1 teaspoon garlic powder

1 teaspoon freshly squeezed lemon juice

1. Preheat the oven to 400°F and line a baking sheet with parchment paper.

2. Combine the potatoes, bell pepper, onion, and green beans in a large bowl and toss with the vegetable broth, garlic powder, and lemon juice.

3. Bake for 25 to 30 minutes, or until the potatoes are fork-tender.

MINI RED POTATOES

RED BELL PEPPER

YELLOW ONION

GREEN BEANS

VEGETABLE BROTH

GARLIC POWDER

LEMON (JUICE)

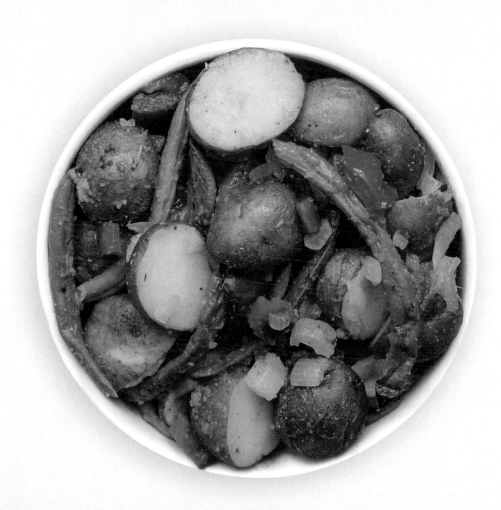

sheet pan roasted vegetables

I love sheet pan recipes because they require very little cleanup and minimal prep. These easy roasted vegetables are no exception. This is a great combo to meal prep each week and have on hand to serve on the side of just about anything!

MAKES 6 servings ✦ **FROM START TO FINISH:** 30 minutes

1½ cups baby carrots

1½ cups Brussels sprouts, chopped

1 medium-size sweet potato, diced but not peeled

1 red onion, diced

5 garlic cloves, peeled and minced

1 teaspoon pure maple syrup

1 teaspoon sea salt

1. Preheat the oven to 400°F and line a baking sheet with parchment paper.

2. Combine all the chopped vegetables in a large bowl and stir in the garlic, maple syrup, and sea salt to coat.

3. Pour the vegetables onto the baking sheet, arrange in a single layer, and bake for 25 to 30 minutes, or until soft.

4. Store in the fridge for up to 4 days.

BABY CARROTS   BRUSSELS SPROUTS   SWEET POTATO   RED ONION   GARLIC (CLOVES)   MAPLE SYRUP

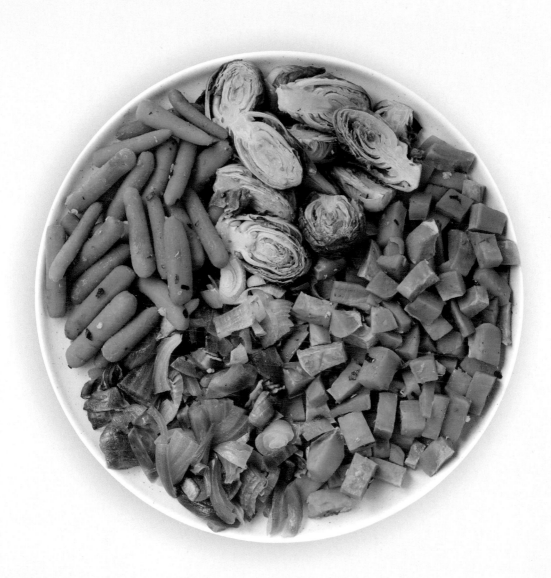

simple sides

plant-
filled
desserts

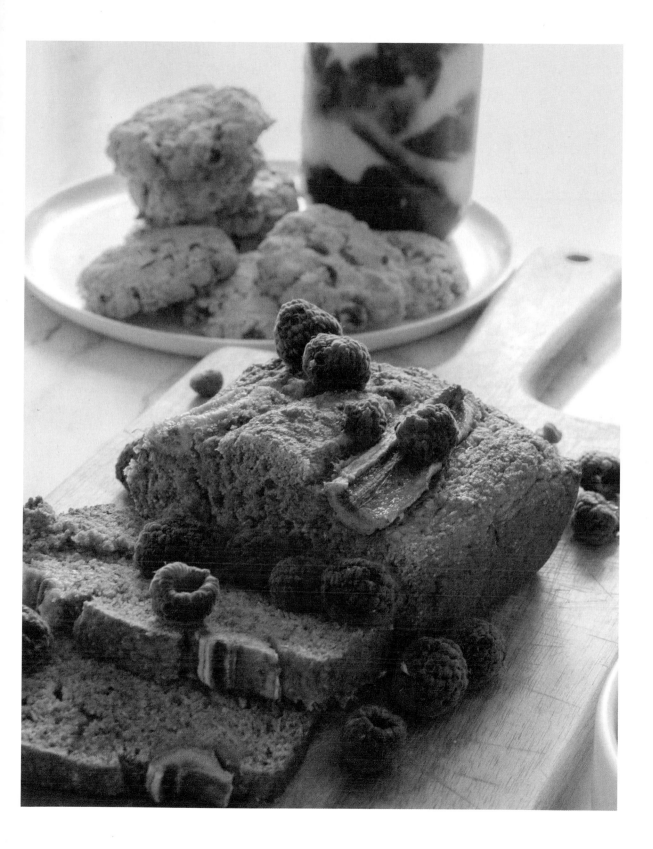

nice cream recipes

Something magical happens when you put frozen fruit in a food processor. It's called nice cream, and it can best be described as a fruit-flavored soft serve. For best results, I suggest peeling your bananas and slicing them into "coins" before freezing. They'll be easier and smoother to blend this way!

notes

For a nut-free version, use oat or soy milk instead.

For a more realistic, scoopable vegan nice cream, transfer to a lidded container and freeze for 2 hours.

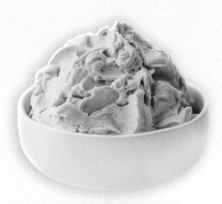

plain banana nice cream
page 240

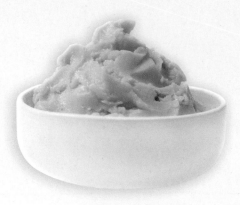

mango nice cream
page 240

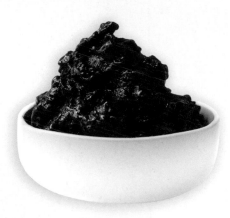

lil raz nice cream
page 241

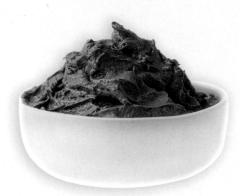

double chocolate nice cream
page 241

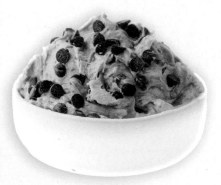

peanut butter chocolate chip nice cream
page 242

plain banana nice cream

MAKES 1 serving ✦ **FROM START TO FINISH:** 5 minutes

2 large bananas, peeled, sliced into coins, and frozen

2 tablespoons unsweetened almond milk

Combine all the ingredients in a food processor with an S blade. Process until a smooth, thick texture is achieved. Serve immediately.

FROZEN BANANA

ALMOND MILK

mango nice cream

MAKES 1 serving ✦ **FROM START TO FINISH:** 5 minutes

2½ cups frozen mango

3 tablespoons unsweetened almond milk

Combine all the ingredients in a food processor with an S blade. Process until a smooth, thick texture is achieved. Serve immediately.

FROZEN MANGO

ALMOND MILK

lil raz nice cream

MAKES 1 serving ✦ **FROM START TO FINISH:** 5 minutes

2½ cups frozen raspberries

3 tablespoons unsweetened almond milk

Combine all the ingredients in a food processor with an S blade. Process until a smooth, thick texture is achieved. Serve immediately.

FROZEN RASPBERRIES

ALMOND MILK

double chocolate nice cream

MAKES 1 serving ✦ **FROM START TO FINISH:** 5 minutes

2 large bananas, peeled, sliced into coins, and frozen

3 tablespoons unsweetened cocoa powder

3 tablespoons unsweetened almond milk

1 teaspoon pure vanilla extract

Combine all the ingredients in a food processor with an S blade. Process until a smooth, thick texture is achieved. Serve immediately.

FROZEN BANANA

COCOA POWDER

ALMOND MILK

VANILLA EXTRACT

peanut butter chocolate chip
nice cream

MAKES 1 serving ✦ **FROM START TO FINISH:** 5 minutes

2 large bananas, peeled, sliced into coins, and frozen

¼ cup all-natural peanut butter

2 tablespoons unsweetened almond milk

2 tablespoons vegan dark chocolate chips

Combine all the ingredients in a food processor with an S blade. Process until a smooth, thick texture is achieved. Fold in chocolate chips and serve immediately.

FROZEN BANANA

PEANUT BUTTER

ALMOND MILK

DARK CHOCOLATE CHIPS

note

For a peanut-free version, use a soy-based peanut butter alternative instead of peanut butter.

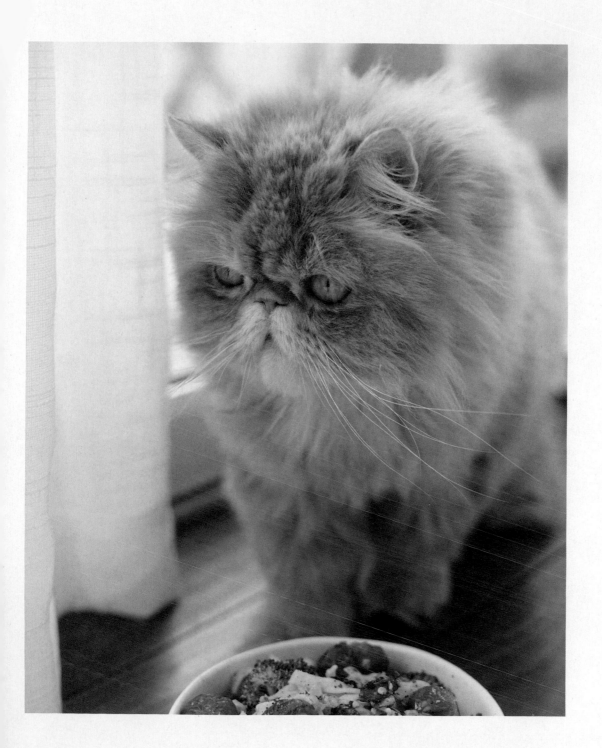

ultimate banana split

This healthy twist on a banana split sees a grilled caramelized banana loaded with creamy coconut yogurt, rolled oats, and a generous topping of mixed berries. It's also a fabulous recipe for kids who can get involved in the assembly and choose their own healthy toppings.

MAKES 1 serving ✦ **FROM START TO FINISH:** 10 minutes

1 banana, sliced in half

1 cup unsweetened coconut yogurt

2 tablespoons rolled oats

½ cup blueberries

½ cup strawberries

1. Place the banana slices, core side down, in a nonstick skillet. Brown over medium heat for about 2 minutes, or until slightly caramelized, then carefully flip and repeat on the other side.

2. Transfer to a serving plate and top with the coconut yogurt, oats, blueberries, and strawberries.

BANANA

COCONUT YOGURT

ROLLED OATS

BLUEBERRIES

STRAWBERRIES

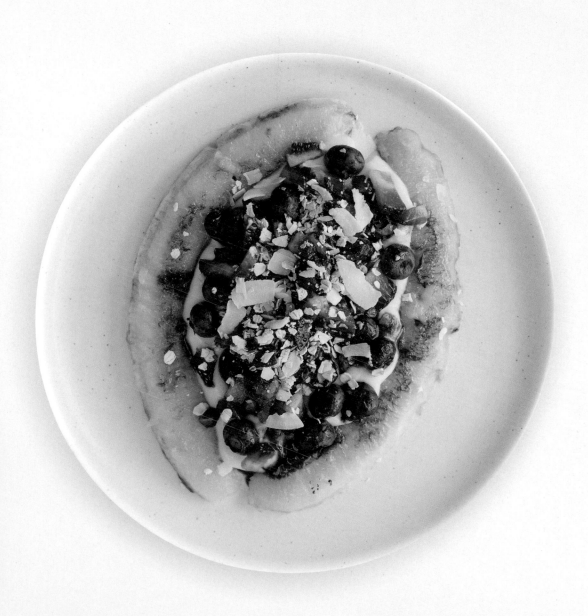

plant-filled desserts

berry galaxy muffins

These muffins remind me of the kind of treat you would see in a bakery display case. Rather than being filled with sugar, they are made with simple, good-for-you ingredients. So good that they could double as breakfast or dessert!

MAKES 8 servings ✦ **FROM START TO FINISH:** 35 minutes

½ cup unsweetened almond milk

¾ cup unsweetened applesauce

¼ cup pure maple syrup

1 teaspoon pure vanilla extract

2½ cups whole wheat flour

½ teaspoon baking soda

½ teaspoon baking powder

½ teaspoon salt

1 cup mixed frozen berries

1. Preheat the oven to 375°F.

2. Mix the almond milk, applesauce, maple syrup, and vanilla in a bowl.

3. In a separate bowl, combine the whole wheat flour, baking soda, baking powder, and salt.

4. Combine the milk mixture with the flour mixture until a smooth batter is formed. Fold in the berries until they are distributed evenly throughout the batter.

5. In a nonstick or lined standard 12-well muffin tin, fill eight muffin wells three-quarters full of the batter.

6. Bake for 25 minutes, or until a toothpick inserted into the center of a muffin comes out clean.

7. Remove from the oven and allow to cool for 15 minutes before serving.

notes

For a nut-free version, swap out the almond milk for oat or soy milk.

For a gluten-free version, replace the whole wheat flour with an all-purpose gluten-free blend.

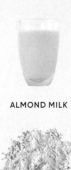

ALMOND MILK

APPLESAUCE

MAPLE SYRUP

VANILLA EXTRACT

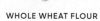

WHOLE WHEAT FLOUR

BAKING SODA

BAKING POWDER

FROZEN BERRIES

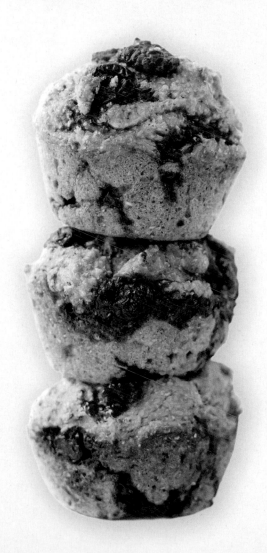

plant-filled desserts

stuffed dates

This is the easiest recipe in my cookbook, but don't pass it by! These simple stuffed dates literally taste like a Twix bar and take less than two minutes to prep.

MAKES 3 servings ✦ **FROM START TO FINISH:** 2 minutes

6 Medjool dates

¼ cup unsweetened almond butter

Flaky sea salt

1. Use a sharp knife to cut lengthwise down the middle of each date. Remove the pit.

2. Add a spoonful of almond butter to the center of each date, and sprinkle with flaky sea salt.

note For a nut-free version, use tahini instead.

DATES

ALMOND BUTTER

FLAKY SALT

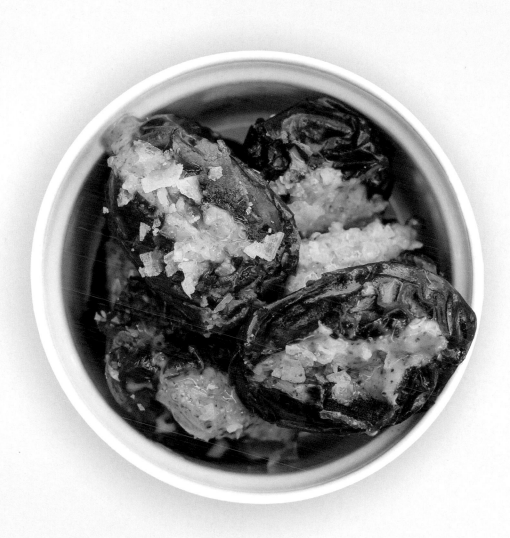

peanut butter thumbprint cookies

I believe the sign of a really good peanut butter cookie is whether it melts in your mouth. These cookies definitely pass the test, and even better, they require just one bowl and four ingredients to whip together.

MAKES 8 servings ✦ **FROM START TO FINISH:** 20 minutes

1 cup all-natural peanut butter

¾ cup oat flour

¼ cup pure maple syrup

4 tablespoons Strawberry Chia Jam (page 264)

1. Preheat the oven to 350°F and line a baking sheet with parchment paper.

2. Combine all the ingredients, except the chia jam, in a bowl. Wet your hands and form into eight balls. Place at least 2 inches apart on the prepared pan. Flatten the balls with your hands or the back of a fork until they are about 1 inch thick.

3. Softly press a finger into the middle of each cookie to make space for the jam, not pressing all the way through to the pan, and scoop 1½ teaspoons of the jam into each space.

4. Bake for 8 to 10 minutes, or until golden brown.

note For a peanut-free version, use a soy-based peanut butter alternative instead of peanut butter.

PEANUT BUTTER

OAT FLOUR

MAPLE SYRUP

STRAWBERRY CHIA JAM

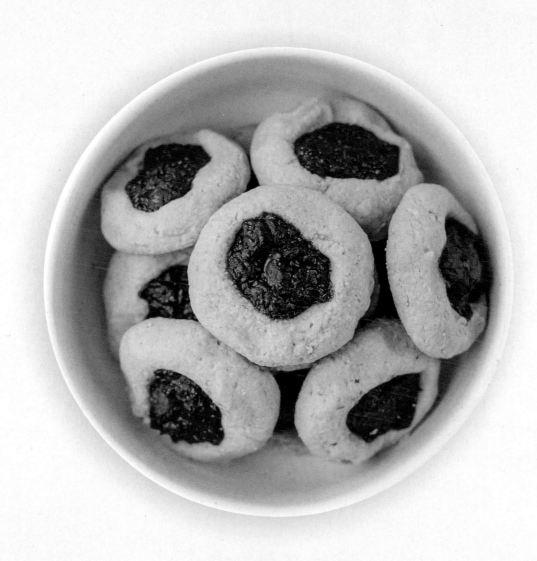

plant-filled desserts

tahini chocolate chip cookies

These are the best cookies that have ever come out of my oven. The combination of drippy, slightly bitter tahini with dark chocolate and flaky salt, all in the vessel of a firm, sweet oat flour batter, is hard to top. Just try not to eat all the raw dough before you bake them.

MAKES 8 to 10 cookies ✦ **FROM START TO FINISH:** 22 minutes

½ cup tahini (drippy, not dry)

⅓ cup pure maple syrup

1 teaspoon pure vanilla extract

1 cup oat flour

½ teaspoon baking powder

¼ cup vegan dark chocolate chips

Flaky salt, for sprinkling

1. Preheat the oven to 400°F and line a baking sheet with parchment paper.

2. Combine the tahini, maple syrup, and vanilla in a large bowl.

3. In a medium-size bowl, mix the oat flour and baking powder. Sift the flour mixture into the tahini mixture and stir until incorporated.

4. Stir in the chocolate chips, then scoop 2-tablespoon-size balls of dough, at least 2 inches apart, onto the prepared baking sheet. The dough will make about 8 large cookies.

5. Using your hands or a fork, squish down each cookie into a ½-inch-thick disk. Top with more chocolate chips and sprinkle with flaky salt.

6. Bake for about 12 minutes, or until golden brown.

TAHINI

MAPLE SYRUP

VANILLA EXTRACT

OAT FLOUR

BAKING POWDER

DARK CHOCOLATE CHIPS

FLAKY SALT

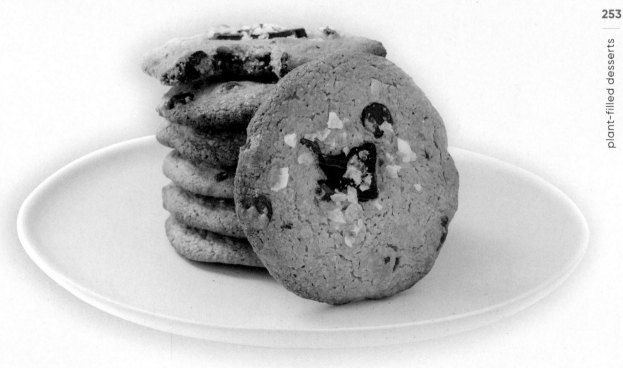

chickpea cookie dough

You might be wondering how it's possible to transform chickpeas into a mouthwatering raw cookie dough. Instead of asking questions, just try it and prepare to have your mind blown by all the cookie goodness. Remember, this is a treat meant to be enjoyed raw. I've tried baking it and the results are just mediocre.

MAKES 4 servings ✦ **FROM START TO FINISH:** 10 minutes

1 (15-ounce) can chickpeas (about 1½ cups), drained and rinsed

½ cup all-natural peanut butter

¼ cup pure maple syrup

1 teaspoon pure vanilla extract

2 tablespoons rolled oats

Pinch of sea salt

½ cup vegan dark chocolate chips

1. Combine all the ingredients, except the chocolate chips, in a food processor and process until a smooth batter is formed.

2. Transfer to a bowl and fold in the chocolate chips. Enjoy as is.

note

For a peanut-free version, use a soy-based peanut butter alternative or tahini instead of peanut butter.

CHICKPEAS

PEANUT BUTTER

MAPLE SYRUP

VANILLA
EXTRACT

ROLLED OATS

DARK
CHOCOLATE
CHIPS

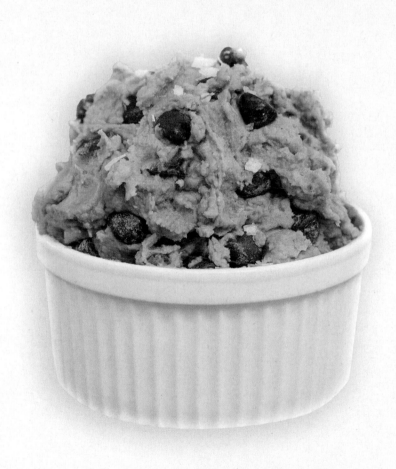

peach crumble

This crumble screams "summer" with farm-fresh juicy peaches and a cinnamon-spiced oat topping. It's also downright addicting, especially when served with coconut whipped cream or yogurt.

MAKES 6 servings ✦ **FROM START TO FINISH:** 40 minutes

PEACH BASE
7 peaches, pitted and sliced

1½ tablespoons pure maple syrup

1½ teaspoons ground cinnamon, Ceylon if possible

1 tablespoon cornstarch or arrowroot powder

Pinch of salt

CRUMBLE
1½ cups rolled oats

½ cup oat flour

¼ cup pure maple syrup

1½ teaspoons ground cinnamon, Ceylon if possible

Pinch of salt

1. Preheat the oven to 375°F.

2. **Prepare the peach base:** In a 9 x 9-inch baking dish, combine the peach slices, maple syrup, cinnamon, cornstarch, and salt. Mix until the peaches are evenly coated.

3. **Prepare the crumble topping:** Combine the oats, oat flour, maple syrup, cinnamon, and salt. Pour on top of the peach mixture until evenly dispersed.

4. Bake for 30 minutes, or until golden and bubbly. Remove from the oven and allow to cool for 5 minutes to set before serving.

notes

Pairs well with unsweetened coconut yogurt, Plain Banana Nice Cream (page 240), or store-bought coconut whipped cream.

You can use frozen peaches for this recipe. Just allow them to thaw first, and drain the excess liquid.

PEACH

MAPLE SYRUP

CINNAMON

CORNSTARCH

ROLLED OATS

OAT FLOUR

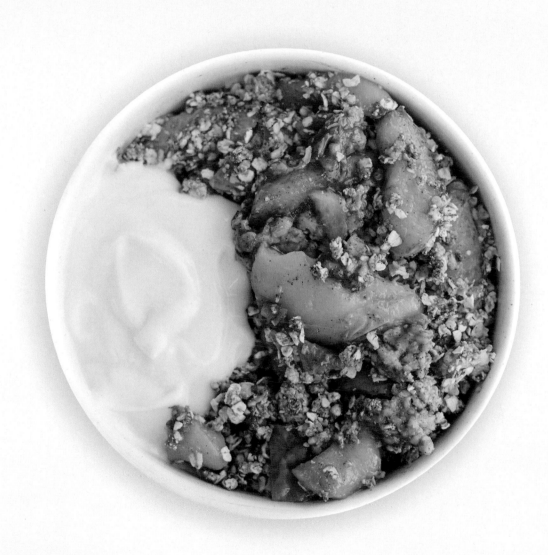

perfect chocolate pudding

As a kid, I had an obsession with Jell-O chocolate pudding cups. I'd sneak at least two into my lunch bag every day and be hyped up on sugar until bedtime. I still get a chocolate pudding craving now and again, and this pudding made with chia seeds hits the spot every time.

MAKES 4 servings ✦ **FROM START TO FINISH:** 5 minutes

2 cups unsweetened almond milk

6 Medjool dates, pitted and soaked for 20 minutes

6 tablespoons chia seeds

¼ cup unsweetened cocoa powder

1. Combine all the ingredients in a high-speed blender or food processor and process until completely smooth.

note For a nut-free version, use oat or soy milk instead.

ALMOND MILK

DATES

CHIA SEEDS

COCOA POWDER

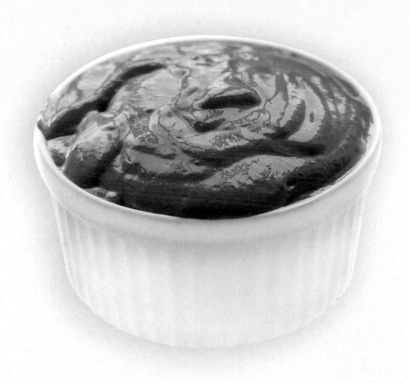

mini vegan raspberry cheeze cakes

These mini cheeze cakes are a beautiful, rich, and delicious no-bake recipe made with soaked cashews. The secret to the cheesy flavor is adding nutritional yeast to the cashew filling. In individual servings, these mini cheeze cakes are the perfect recipe to make if you want to wow your friends and family with a decadent vegan dessert.

MAKES 8 servings   ✦   **FROM START TO FINISH:** 4 hours and 10 minutes

CRUST
⅓ cup Medjool dates, pitted
¾ cup rolled oats
¾ tablespoon unsweetened almond milk, plus more as needed to combine

CAKE BATTER
3 cups raw cashews, soaked in water overnight and drained
⅓ cup unsweetened almond milk

⅓ cup pure maple syrup
2 teaspoons nutritional yeast
1 teaspoon pure vanilla extract
½ teaspoon freshly squeezed lemon juice
Pinch of salt
½ cup frozen raspberries, plus more for topping (optional)

1. Line eight wells of a standard muffin tin with silicone or paper liners.

2. **Prepare the crust:** Combine the dates, rolled oats, and almond milk in a food processor and process until smooth.

3. Place a spoonful of the crust mixture in each of the eight lined muffin wells, pressing down with your figures to create a solid base for the cheeze cakes.

4. **Now, make the cake batter:** Combine all the batter ingredients, except the raspberries, in a high-speed blender and blend until completely smooth. Once a velvety consistency is achieved, pour the raspberries into the blender cup and use a spoon or spatula to disperse them throughout the batter.

5. Transfer the batter into a piping bag, or a resealable plastic bag with a small hole sliced off a bottom corner, and squeeze the batter into the eight crust-filled muffin wells. Top with additional raspberries, if desired, and place the cakes in the freezer for 4 hours.

6. These are best enjoyed when frozen, then thawed in the refrigerator for 15 minutes before eating.

DATES

ROLLED OATS

ALMOND MILK

CASHEWS

MAPLE SYRUP

NUTRITIONAL YEAST

VANILLA EXTRACT

LEMON (JUICE)

FROZEN RASPBERRIES

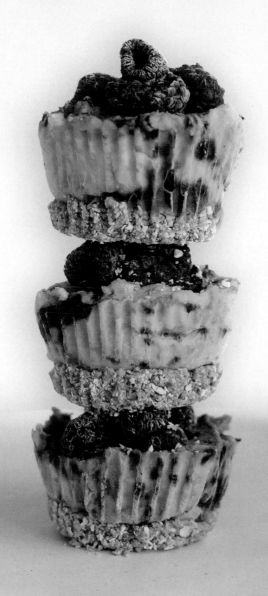

plant-filled desserts

one-bowl pumpkin banana bread

This loaf is dangerous. Friends and family have reported that even though it serves eight, it magically disappears within twenty-four hours. Something about the combination of the earthy pumpkin, sweet banana, and dark chocolate chips throws this one right over the edge!

MAKES 8 servings ✦ **FROM START TO FINISH:** 50 minutes

2½ bananas, mashed (about 1½ cups)

½ cup pure pumpkin puree (not pumpkin pie filling)

½ cup pure maple syrup

1 teaspoon pure vanilla extract

1 teaspoon pumpkin pie spice or ground cinnamon

1½ cups whole wheat flour

1 teaspoon baking soda

½ teaspoon baking powder

¼ cup ground flaxseeds

Pinch of sea salt

½ cup vegan dark chocolate chips (optional)

1. Preheat the oven to 350°F and line an 8½ x 4½-inch loaf pan with parchment paper.

2. Place the bananas in a large bowl, and using the back of a fork or a potato masher, crush them until you achieve a puree. Add the pumpkin puree, maple syrup, and vanilla to the bowl and mix until fully combined.

3. Add the rest of the ingredients, except the chocolate chips, and gently stir. You want to make sure not to overmix, or it will result in a glutinous loaf. The mixture should resemble pancake batter.

4. Stir in the chocolate chips, holding back 1 tablespoon for topping. Pour the mixture into the prepared loaf pan and top with the remaining chocolate chips.

5. Bake for 50 minutes, or until a toothpick inserted into the center comes out clean. Remove from the oven and allow to cool to room temperature before slicing.

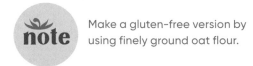

note Make a gluten-free version by using finely ground oat flour.

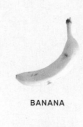

BANANA

PUMPKIN PUREE

MAPLE SYRUP

VANILLA EXTRACT

PUMPKIN PIE SPICE

WHOLE WHEAT FLOUR

BAKING SODA

BAKING POWDER

GROUND FLAXSEEDS

DARK CHOCOLATE
CHIPS (OPTIONAL)

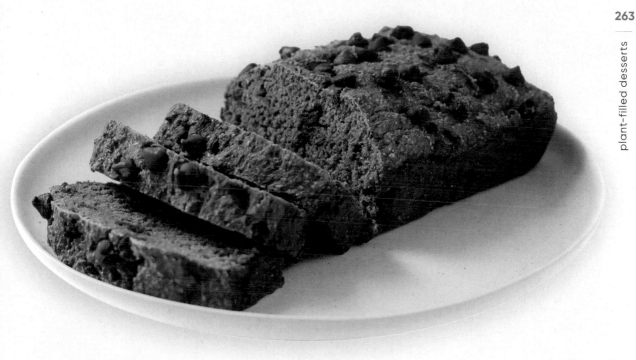

strawberry chia jam

Who knew that the same little seeds you use to grow a beard in your terra-cotta garden gnome could have amazing jam-making superpowers? This jam is so easy, you'll never buy it from a grocery store again! This recipe is extremely versatile and can work with other berries, such as raspberries, blueberries, and blackberries, or mixed frozen fruit as well. I suggest storing it in an 8-ounce mason jar.

MAKES 6 servings ✦ **FROM START TO FINISH:** 10 minutes

2 cups sliced fresh strawberries

1 tablespoon pure maple syrup

2 tablespoons chia seeds

1. Place the strawberries and maple syrup in a saucepan. Cover and cook over medium heat for 6 to 8 minutes, or until the strawberries are soft.

2. Once the strawberries are soft, crush them with a fork until you achieve an applesauce-like consistency.

3. Remove from the heat and let cool, then transfer the strawberry mixture to a jar.

4. Add the chia seeds and mix. Let the jam sit for a couple of minutes before serving.

5. The jam will become more "jammy" after refrigeration. Store in the fridge for up to 5 days.

STRAWBERRIES   MAPLE SYRUP   CHIA SEEDS

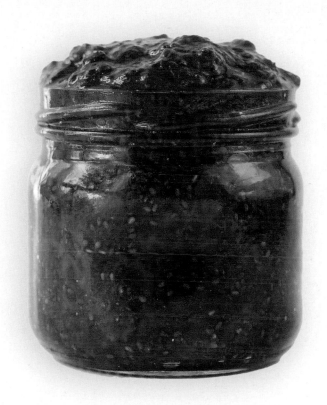

fudgy avocado brownies

Prepare to lick the spatula clean with these delicious fudgy brownies. By combining creamy avocado with whole wheat flour, maple syrup, and cocoa powder, you're left with a rich chocolate batter that makes the fudgiest brownies in the world. If you have some skeptical friends and family, fear not; the avocado is completely undetectable in this sweet treat.

MAKES 16 servings ✦ **FROM START TO FINISH:** 50 minutes

1 ripe avocado, peeled, pitted, and mashed

¾ cup unsweetened almond milk

½ cup pure maple syrup

1 cup whole wheat flour

½ cup unsweetened cocoa powder

1 teaspoon baking soda

½ teaspoon sea salt

½ cup vegan dark chocolate chips

1. Preheat the oven to 350°F and line an 8 x 8-inch baking pan with parchment paper.

2. Combine the mashed avocado, almond milk, and maple syrup in a large bowl.

3. In a separate bowl, combine the whole wheat flour, cocoa powder, baking soda, and sea salt.

4. Mix the flour mixture into the avocado mixture until a smooth batter is formed. Fold in the chocolate chips. Pour the batter evenly into the prepared pan.

5. Bake for 40 minutes, or until a fork poked into the center comes out clean. Remove from the oven and let the brownies sit for 15 minutes before cutting.

AVOCADO

ALMOND MILK

MAPLE SYRUP

WHOLE WHEAT FLOUR

COCOA POWDER

BAKING SODA

DARK CHOCOLATE
CHIPS

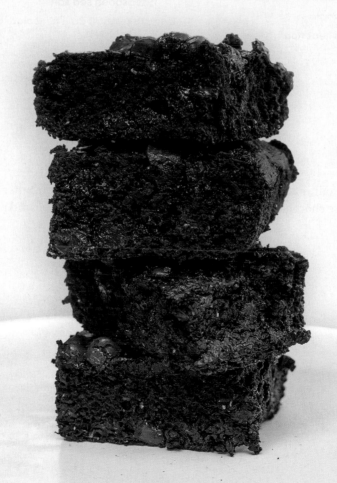

hot bevvies

Few things are more comforting than a warm mug between your hands. Whether we're talking about a matcha latte or cocoa, hot bevvies are an amazing way to start and end your day in peace. Here are four of my favorites.

 For a nut-free version, use oat milk instead.

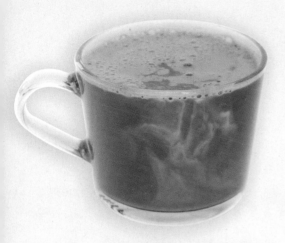

winter eve hot cocoa
page 270

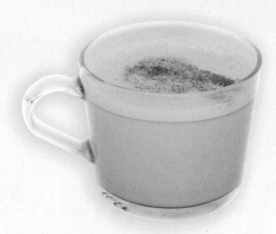

good night turmeric latte
page 271

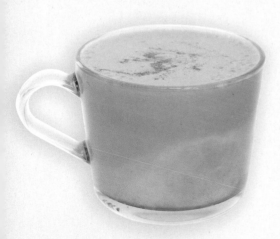

matcha green tea latte
page 272

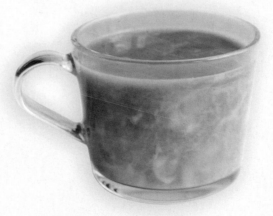

pumpkin pie latte
page 273

winter eve hot cocoa

MAKES 1 serving ✦ **FROM START TO FINISH:** 5 minutes

2 cups unsweetened cashew milk

2 tablespoons unsweetened cocoa powder

1½ tablespoons pure maple syrup

1. Whisk together all the ingredients in a saucepan.

2. Bring to a boil over high heat, then lower the heat to a slow simmer and stir constantly until the cocoa powder has dissolved completely. Pour in a mug and enjoy.

CASHEW MILK

COCOA POWDER

MAPLE SYRUP

good night turmeric latte

MAKES 1 serving ✦ **FROM START TO FINISH:** 5 minutes

1½ cups unsweetened almond milk

½ teaspoon ground turmeric

½ teaspoon ground cinnamon, Ceylon if possible

½ teaspoon pure vanilla extract

1 teaspoon pure maple syrup

Pinch of freshly ground black pepper

1. Whisk together all the ingredients in a saucepan.

2. Bring to a boil over high heat, then lower the heat to a slow simmer and stir constantly until the spices have dissolved completely. Pour in a mug and enjoy.

ALMOND MILK

TURMERIC

CINNAMON

VANILLA EXTRACT

MAPLE SYRUP

notes

Adding a pinch of black pepper to this turmeric latte helps activate the curcumin in the turmeric, which has amazing anti-inflammatory benefits.

If you're unfamiliar with a turmeric latte, this is not an overly sweet drink. It has a soul-warming, light but slightly bitter flavor from the cinnamon, turmeric, and black pepper.

matcha green tea latte

MAKES 1 serving ✦ **FROM START TO FINISH:** 5 minutes

1½ cups unsweetened cashew milk

1½ teaspoons matcha powder, ceremonial grade if possible

1 date, pitted

Pinch of ground cinnamon

1. Combine all the ingredients in a blender and blend until smooth.

2. Transfer to a small saucepan and heat over high heat until warm. Pour in a mug and enjoy.

CASHEW MILK

MATCHA

DATES

CINNAMON

note

The quality of matcha can vary greatly. Look for matcha powder that is a deep green color rather than light, and that is ceremonial grade if possible.

pumpkin pie latte

MAKES 1 serving ✦ **FROM START TO FINISH:** 5 minutes

⅔ cup brewed coffee

2 tablespoons pure pumpkin puree (not pumpkin pie filling)

1 cup unsweetened cashew milk

½ teaspoon pumpkin pie spice or ground cinnamon

1 tablespoon pure maple syrup

1. Whisk together all the ingredients in a saucepan.

2. Bring to a boil over high heat, then lower the heat to a slow simmer and stir constantly until the spices have dissolved completely. Pour in a mug and enjoy.

BREWED COFFEE

PUMPKIN PUREE

CASHEW MILK

PUMPKIN PIE SPICE

MAPLE SYRUP

plant-filled desserts

recipe nutritional information

I calculated these nutritionals with the recipes as written (without extra toppings and as the ingredients are listed, rather than with swaps). Of course, your ingredients may differ—as I mentioned earlier, some ingredients have different components. One almond milk may have more protein and higher fat and calories than another. But these should be good, basic guidelines if you are interested in your macros!

Plant-Filled Mornings

Overnight Oats & Breakfast Puddings

Banana Walnut Explosion
Calories: 308, Fat: 12 g, Carbs: 46 g, Fiber: 9.2 g, Protein: 10 g

Midnight Chocolate Cherry
Calories: 406, Fat: 14 g, Carbs: 65 g, Fiber: 12 g, Protein: 11 g

Antioxidant Oat Cups
Calories: 261, Fat: 7 g, Carbs: 42 g, Fiber: 10 g, Protein: 8 g

PB & Jelly
Calories: 305, Fat: 13 g, Carbs: 41 g, Fiber: 8 g, Protein: 10 g

Chocolate Chip Cookie Dough
Calories: 351, Fat: 11 g, Carbs: 53 g, Fiber: 6 g, Protein: 7 g

Granny's Apple Pie
Calories: 364, Fat: 8 g, Carbs: 68 g, Fiber: 11 g, Protein: 8 g

Coo-Coo for Coconuts Chia Pudding
Calories: 316, Fat: 21 g, Carbs: 27 g, Fiber: 14 g, Protein: 9 g

Flaxmeal Pudding
Calories: 272, Fat: 10 g, Carbs: 40 g, Fiber: 9 g, Protein: 8 g

Banana Stovetop Oats
Calories: 295, Fat: 6 g, Carbs: 57 g, Fiber: 9 g, Protein: 8 g

Superseed Muesli
Calories: 189, Fat: 9 g, Carbs: 22 g, Fiber: 7 g, Protein: 6 g

Bravocado Toast
Calories: 220, Fat: 12 g, Carbs: 23 g, Fiber: 8 g, Protein: 6 g

Sunshine Scramble
Calories: 209, Fat: 12 g, Carbs: 7 g, Fiber: 4 g, Protein: 24 g

Blueberry Lemon Pancakes
Calories: 193, Fat: 2 g, Carbs: 38 g, Fiber: 6 g, Protein: 6 g

Cowboy Casanova Breakfast Hash
Calories: 336, Fat: 0 g, Carbs: 74 g, Fiber: 13 g, Protein: 13 g

Tempeh Bacon
Calories: 156, Fat: 6 g, Carbs: 15 g, Fiber: 5 g, Protein: 11 g

Welcome to Smoothie Land
MEAN GREEN SMOOTHIES
The Starter
Calories: 210, Fat: 9 g, Carbs: 30 g, Fiber: 5 g, Protein: 7 g

The Big Glow
Calories: 225, Fat: 8 g, Carbs: 35 g, Fiber: 11 g, Protein: 6 g

Minty Mojito
Calories: 171, Fat: 0 g, Carbs: 44 g, Fiber: 8 g, Protein: 4 g

Hulk Smoothie
Calories: 208, Fat: 5 g, Carbs: 32 g, Fiber: 6 g, Protein: 11 g

Par Slay
Calories: 395, Fat: 8 g, Carbs: 78 g, Fiber: 17 g, Protein: 9 g

Good Gut
Calories: 252, Fat: 12 g, Carbs: 36 g, Fiber: 9 g, Protein: 7 g

FRUIT-FILLED WONDERS
Piña Colada
Calories: 199, Fat: 11 g, Carbs: 25 g, Fiber: 4 g, Protein: 5 g

Pink Elephant
Calories: 298, Fat: 16 g, Carbs: 36 g, Fiber: 12 g, Protein: 9 g

Mango Tango
Calories: 214, Fat: 9 g, Carbs: 32 g, Fiber: 5 g, Protein: 2 g

Peach Cobbler Smoothie
Calories: 279, Fat: 8 g, Carbs: 53 g, Fiber: 9 g, Protein: 7 g

Blueberry Fields
Calories: 308, Fat: 10 g, Carbs: 54 g, Fiber: 11 g, Protein: 5 g

Banana Mama
Calories: 342, Fat: 15 g, Carbs: 48 g, Fiber: 16 g, Protein: 7 g

DECADENT SMOOTHIES
Ice Capp
Calories: 127, Fat: 2 g, Carbs: 28 g, Fiber: 4 g, Protein: 2 g

Watermelon High Slushy
Calories: 96, Fat: 0 g, Carbs: 25 g, Fiber: 1 g, Protein: 2 g

Snickers Smoothie
Calories: 340, Fat: 19 g, Carbs: 40 g, Fiber: 10 g, Protein: 11 g

Red Velvet
Calories: 210, Fat: 5 g, Carbs: 42 g, Fiber: 12 g, Protein: 5 g

Pumpkin Pie
Calories: 307, Fat: 2 g, Carbs: 72 g, Fiber: 10 g, Protein: 5 g

Cake Batter
Calories: 297, Fat: 5 g, Carbs: 62 g,
Fiber: 7 g, Protein: 6 g

Breakfast Cookies

Chocolate Chip Banana Bread Breakfast Cookies
Nutritional information per cookie.
Calories 130, Fat: 4 g, Carbs: 23 g,
Fiber: 3 g, Protein: 3 g

Dreamy Zucchini Breakfast Cookies
Nutritional information per cookie.
Calories: 130, Fat: 7 g, Carbs: 15 g,
Fiber: 3 g, Protein: 4 g

Pumpkin Breakfast Cookies
Nutritional information per cookie.
Calories: 214, Fat: 6 g, Carbs: 36 g,
Fiber: 3 g, Protein: 4 g

Nutrient Bomb Breakfast Cookies
Nutritional information per cookie.
Calories: 177, Fat: 6 g, Carbs: 30 g,
Fiber: 5 g, Protein: 5 g

Souper Bowls

Belly-Warming Minestrone Soup
Nutritional information per serving
based on 4 servings: Calories: 314,
Fat: 1 g, Carbs: 63 g, Fiber: 15 g,
Protein: 13 g

Wicked Red Curry Soup
Calories: 166, Fat: 6 g, Carbs: 23 g,
Fiber: 5 g, Protein: 4 g

Roasted Red Pepper & Cauliflower Soup
Calories: 198, Fat: 8 g, Carbs: 27 g,
Fiber: 7 g, Protein: 8 g

Butternut Squash Soup
Nutritional information per serving
based on 4 servings: Calories: 211,
Fat: 6 g, Carbs: 38 g, Fiber: 5 g,
Protein: 3 g

Fresh Tomato Red Lentil Bisque
Nutritional information per serving
based on 4 servings: Calories: 273,
Fat: 1 g, Carbs: 51 g, Fiber: 14 g,
Protein: 17 g

In a Jiffy Tomato Soup
Calories: 165, Fat: 4 g, Carbs: 26 g,
Fiber: 8 g, Protein: 5 g

Lazy Lentil Soup
Nutritional information per serving
based on 6 servings: Calories: 328,
Fat: 1 g, Carbs: 63 g, Fiber:
18 g, Protein: 19 g

Broccoli Chedda' Soup
Nutritional information per serving
based on 4 servings: Calories:
203, Fat: 8 g, Carbs: 29 g, Fiber:
6 g, Protein: 8 g

Wild Rice & Lemon Soup
Calories: 142, Fat: 2 g, Carbs: 28 g,
Fiber: 4 g, Protein: 5 g

"Not Your College" Ramen
Without toppings: Calories: 370,
Fat: 15 g, Carbs: 44 g, Fiber: 5 g,
Protein: 16 g

Chickpea Noodle Soup
Calories: 320, Fat: 3 g, Carbs: 63 g,
Fiber: 8 g, Protein: 9 g

Creamy Potato Leek Soup
Nutritional information per serving
based on 4 servings: Calories:
200, Fat: 1.8 g, Carbs: 38.6 g,
Fiber: 3.4 g, Protein, 9.5 g

Magical Mineral Broth
Nutritional information per serving
based on 15 servings: Calories:
33, Fat: 0 g, Carbs: 8 g, Fiber: 2 g,
Protein: 1 g

Sammys + Salads

Superloaded Veggie Wrap
Calories: 511, Fat: 16 g, Carbs: 78 g,
Fiber: 12 g, Protein: 20 g

Smashed Chickpea Salad Sandwich
Calories: 438, Fat: 15 g, Carbs:
57 g, Fiber: 12 g, Protein: 18 g

TLT (Tempeh, Lettuce, Tomato)
Calories: 465, Fat: 12 g, Carbs:
70 g, Fiber: 3 g, Protein: 24 g

Buffalo Chick'n Wrap
Calories: 503, Fat: 16 g, Carbs:
67 g, Fiber: 10 g, Protein: 26 g

Garden of Life Pita Pizza
Calories: 464, Fat: 23 g, Carbs:
55 g, Fiber: 9 g, Protein: 16 g

Build-a-Bowl
Calories: 724, Fat: 43 g, Carbs:
72 g, Fiber: 19 g, Protein: 27 g

Beaming Burrito Bowl
Calories: 430, Fat: 18 g, Carbs:
72 g, Fiber: 17 g, Protein: 19 g

Tangy Potato Salad
Calories: 228, Fat: 3 g, Carbs: 46 g,
Fiber: 10 g, Protein: 9 g

Balsamic Pasta Salad
Calories: 341, Fat: 9 g, Carbs: 59 g,
Fiber: 5 g, Protein: 6 g

Crunchy Peanut Shredded Salad
Calories: 364, Fat: 15 g, Carbs:
47 g, Fiber: 8 g, Protein: 15 g

Cool Ranch Kale Salad
Calories: 213, Fat: 6 g, Carbs: 28 g,
Fiber: 10 g, Protein: 16 g

Citrus Solstice Salad
Calories: 171, Fat: 7 g, Carbs: 23 g,
Fiber: 5 g, Protein: 5 g

Quinoa Cranberry Harvest Salad
Calories: 288, Fat: 5.9 g, Carbs: 54 g,
Fiber: 5.6 g, Protein: 8.4 g

Roasted Corn, Bell Pepper & Cilantro Salad
Calories: 354, Fat: 16 g, Carbs:
50 g, Fiber: 11 g, Protein: 8 g

The Main Event

Presto Pesto Penne
Calories: 562, Fat: 19 g, Carbs:
90 g, Fiber: 14 g, Protein: 22 g

Garlic Lovers' Vegan Alfredo
Calories: 513, Fat: 3 g, Carbs:
104 g, Fiber: 17 g, Protein: 24 g

Creamy Mushroom Pasta
Calories: 654, Fat: 18 g, Carbs:
107 g, Fiber: 9 g, Protein: 24 g

Garden Bolognese
Calories: 533, Fat: 3 g, Carbs:
108 g, Fiber: 19 g, Protein: 23 g

Ginger Garlic Noodz
Calories: 279, Fat: 6 g, Carbs: 49 g,
Fiber: 8 g, Protein: 8 g

Sheet Pan Fajitas
Calories: 217, Fat: 3 g, Carbs: 43 g,
Fiber: 3 g, Protein: 7 g

The Big Boss Burrito
Calories including all toppings listed: 631, Fat: 21 g, Carbs: 96 g, Fiber: 19 g, Protein: 18 g

10-Minute Tacos
Caloric information excludes suggested toppings: Calories: 272, Fat: 14 g, Carbs: 31 g, Fiber: 4 g, Protein: 7 g

Rainbow Summer Rolls
Calories: 249, Fat: 3 g, Carbs: 53 g, Fiber: 3 g, Protein: 4 g

Staple Tempeh Stir-Fry
Calories: 424, Fat: 8 g, Carbs: 66 g, Fiber: 9.5 g, Protein: 20 g

Simple Peanut Sauce Stir-Fry
Calories: 389, Fat: 11 g, Carbs: 57 g, Fiber: 5 g, Protein: 19 g

Plant-Packed Pad Thai
Calories: 615, Fat: 9 g, Carbs: 114 g, Fiber: 5 g, Protein: 19 g

Pineapple Cauliflower Fried Rice
Calories: 183, Fat: 1 g, Carbs: 37 g, Fiber: 9 g, Protein: 11 g

Hoisin Broccoli Spicy Rice
Calories: 230, Fat: 1 g, Carbs: 49 g, Fiber: 5 g, Protein: 6 g

Sweet 'n' Spicy Tofu Skewers
Calories: 163, Fat: 5 g, Carbs: 19 g, Fiber: 3 g, Protein: 15 g

"Butter" Chickpeas
Calories: 505, Fat: 19 g, Carbs: 70 g, Fiber: 9.5 g, Protein: 15 g

"Everything but the Kitchen Sink" Curry
Calories: 533, Fat: 21 g, Carbs: 76 g, Fiber: 12 g, Protein: 13 g

"Can't Believe It's Vegan" Lasagna
Calories: 378, Fat: 8 g, Carbs: 62 g, Fiber: 7 g, Protein: 17 g

Irish Stew Without the Beef or Booze
Calories: 311, Fat: 1 g, Carbs: 67 g, Fiber: 9 g, Protein: 10 g

Golden Shepherd's Pie
Calories: 193, Fat: 1 g, Carbs: 43 g, Fiber: 6 g, Protein: 7 g

BBQ Chickpea Stuffed Sweet Potatoes
Calories: 422, Fat: 11 g, Carbs: 38 g, Fiber: 6 g, Protein: 8 g

Hearty Bean & Sweet Potato Chili
Nutritional information per serving based on 4 servings, garnishes not included: Calories: 395, Fat: 10 g, Carbs: 59 g, Fiber: 21 g, Protein: 20 g

Portobello Mushroom Steaks
Calories: 77, Fat: 0 g, Carbs: 16 g, Fiber: 1 g, Protein: 3 g

Cozy Sweet Potato Peanut Stew
Nutritional information per serving based on 4 servings: Calories: 495, Fat: 17 g, Carbs: 67 g, Fiber: 18 g, Protein: 25 g

Bliss Burgers
Nutritional information for 1 patty with a whole wheat bun, no toppings: Calories: 277, Fat: 3 g, Carbs: 53 g, Fiber: 7 g, Protein: 13 g

Best Ever Cauli Wings
Calories: 221, Fat: 1 g, Carbs: 47 g, Fiber: 4 g, Protein: 6 g

BBQ Jackfruit Pulled Pork
Calories: 327, Fat: 2 g, Carbs: 70 g, Fiber: 11 g, Protein: 9 g

Mac 'n' Peas
Calories: 525, Fat: 2 g, Carbs: 112 g, Fiber: 15 g, Protein: 23 g

Meaty Vegan Lentil Loaf
Calories: 217, Fat: 2 g, Carbs: 40 g, Fiber: 8 g, Protein: 11 g

TGIF Pizza
Calories: 557, Fat: 21 g, Carbs: 75 g, Fiber: 13 g, Protein: 18 g

Let's Get Saucy

Hummus 3 Ways
Garlic Hummus
Calories: 116, Fat: 6 g, Carbs: 12 g, Fiber: 3 g, Protein: 5 g

Beet Hummus
Calories: 122, Fat: 6 g, Carbs: 13 g, Fiber: 3 g, Protein: 5 g

Roasted Red Pepper Hummus
Calories: 98, Fat: 4 g, Carbs: 14 g, Fiber: 3 g, Protein: 4 g

Salad Dressings & Sauces
Go-To Balsamic
Nutritional information per serving based on 4 servings: Calories: 25, Fat: 0 g, Carbs: 6 g, Fiber: 0 g, Protein: 0 g

Apple Cider Vinaigrette
Calories: 12, Fat: 0 g, Carbs: 3 g, Fiber: 0 g, Protein: 0 g

Spicy Peanut Dressing
Calories: 113, Fat: 8 g, Carbs: 8 g, Fiber: 2 g, Protein: 5 g

Classic Tahini Dressing
Calories: 135, Fat: 11 g, Carbs: 8 g, Fiber: 2 g, Protein: 3 g

Turmeric Tahini Dressing
Calories: 124, Fat: 11 g, Carbs: 6 g, Fiber: 2 g, Protein: 3 g

Cilantro Lime Dressing
Nutritional information per serving based on 3 servings: Calories: 86, Fat: 8 g, Carbs: 5 g, Fiber: 4 g, Protein: 1 g

Creamy Ranch Dressing
Nutritional information per serving based on 4 servings: Calories: 59, Fat: 3 g, Carbs: 1 g, Fiber: 0 g, Protein: 6 g

Smokin' BBQ Sauce
Calories based on 4 servings: 102, Fat: 0 g, Carbs: 26 g, Fiber: 1 g, Protein: 1 g

Cashew Mayo
Calories: 60, Fat: 5 g, Carbs: 3 g, Fiber: 1 g, Protein: 2 g

Spinach Basil Pesto
Calories based on 4 servings: 189, Fat: 18 g, Carbs: 7 g, Fiber: 2 g, Protein: 5 g

Easy Vegan Gravy
Calories: 13, Fat: 0 g, Carbs: 3 g, Fiber: 0 g, Protein: 0 g

Vegan Cheeze Sauces
Everything Cheeze Sauce
Calories: 95, Fat: 0 g, Carbs: 20 g, Fiber: 4 g, Protein: 4 g

Vegan Mozzarella
Nutritional information per serving based on 4 servings. Calories: 131, Fat: 10 g, Carbs: 8 g, Fiber: 1 g, Protein: 4 g

Herb & Garlic Cream Cheeze
Calories: 122, Fat: 10 g, Carbs: 7 g, Fiber: 1 g, Protein: 4 g

Vegan Queso
Nutritional information per serving based on 4 servings: Calories: 113, Fat: 7 g, Carbs: 10 g, Fiber: 3 g, Protein: 3 g

Tofu Ricotta
Nutritional information per serving based on 4 servings: Calories: 121, Fat: 5 g, Carbs: 7 g, Fiber: 1 g, Protein: 12 g

Salsas

Mango Salsa
Calories: 134, Fat: 8 g, Carbs: 18 g, Fiber: 5 g, Protein: 2 g

Guacamole
Calories: 168, Fat: 15 g, Carbs: 11 g, Fiber: 7 g, Protein: 3 g

Pico de Gallo
Calories: 33, Fat: 1 g, Carbs: 7 g, Fiber: 2 g, Protein: 2 g

Classic Homemade Salsa
Calories: 61, Fat: 0 g, Carbs: 11 g, Fiber: 3 g, Protein: 3 g

Simple Sides

Golden Mashed Potatoes
Calories: 114, Fat: 0 g, Carbs: 27 g, Fiber: 2 g, Protein: 3 g

Crispy Dill French Fries
Calories: 110, Fat: 0 g, Carbs: 26 g, Fiber: 3 g, Protein: 2 g

Quick Pickled Red Onions
Calories: 15, Fat: 0 g, Carbs: 4 g, Fiber: 1 g, Protein: 0 g

Garlic Asparagus with Cheeze Sauce
Calories: 71, Fat: 0 g, Carbs: 15 g, Fiber: 4 g, Protein: 4 g

Curried Bok Choy
Calories: 53, Fat: 3 g, Carbs: 7 g, Fiber: 2 g, Protein: 2 g

Roasted Baby Potatoes & Green Beans
Calories: 194, Fat: 3 g, Carbs: 43 g, Fiber: 6 g, Protein: 6 g

Sheet Pan Roasted Vegetables
Calories: 55, Fat: 0 g, Carbs: 13 g, Fiber: 3 g, Protein: 2 g

Plant-Filled Desserts

Nice Cream Recipes

Plain Banana Nice Cream
Calories: 246, Fat: 1 g, Carbs: 62 g, Fiber: 7 g, Protein: 3 g

Mango Nice Cream
Calories: 232, Fat: 2 g, Carbs: 53 g, Fiber: 5 g, Protein: 3 g

Lil Raz Nice Cream
Calories: 182, Fat: 3 g, Carbs: 43 g, Fiber: 23 g, Protein: 5 g

Double Chocolate Nice Cream
Calories: 321, Fat: 3 g, Carbs: 72 g, Fiber: 10 g, Protein: 6 g

Peanut Butter Chocolate Chip Nice Cream
Calories: 676, Fat: 35 g, Carbs: 89 g, Fiber: 14 g, Protein: 17 g

Ultimate Banana Split
Calories: 308, Fat: 9.5 g, Carbs: 62 g, Fiber: 15 g, Protein: 4 g

Berry Galaxy Muffins
Calories: 188, Fat: 1 g, Carbs: 38 g, Fiber: 6 g, Protein: 5 g

Stuffed Dates
Calories: 252, Fat: 11 g, Carbs: 38 g, Fiber: 6 g, Protein: 7 g

Peanut Butter Thumbprint Cookies
Calories: 267, Fat: 18 g, Carbs: 24 g, Fiber: 5 g, Protein: 10 g

Tahini Chocolate Chip Cookies
Nutritional information per serving based on 8 servings: Calories: 225, Fat: 12 g, Carbs: 26 g, Fiber: 3 g, Protein: 6 g

Chickpea Cookie Dough
Calories: 486, Fat: 27 g, Carbs: 53 g, Fiber: 11 g, Protein: 16 g

Peach Crumble
Calories: 239, Fat: 3 g, Carbs: 51 g, Fiber: 6 g, Protein: 6 g

Perfect Chocolate Pudding
Calories: 297, Fat: 9 g, Carbs: 73 g, Fiber: 14 g, Protein: 7.5 g

Mini Vegan Raspberry Cheeze Cakes
Calories: 367, Fat: 22 g, Carbs: 37 g, Fiber: 4 g, Protein: 10 g

One-Bowl Pumpkin Banana Bread
Calories: 167, Fat: 3.5 g, Carbs: 33 g, Fiber: 3 g, Protein 3 g

Strawberry Chia Jam
Calories: 48, Fat: 2 g, Carbs: 8 g, Fiber: 3 g, Protein: 1 g

Fudgy Avocado Brownies
Calories: 120, Fat: 4 g, Carbs: 18 g, Fiber: 3 g, Protein: 2 g

Hot Bevvies

Winter Eve Hot Cocoa
Calories: 172, Fat: 5 g, Carbs: 29 g, Fiber: 2 g, Protein: 4 g

Good Night Turmeric Latte
Calories: 87, Fat: 5 g, Carbs: 9 g, Fiber: 3 g, Protein: 2 g

Matcha Green Tea Latte
Calories: 123, Fat: 3 g, Carbs: 21 g, Fiber: 4 g, Protein: 4 g

Pumpkin Pie Latte
Calories: 97, Fat: 2 g, Carbs: 18 g, Fiber: 1 g, Protein: 2 g

acknowledgments

It seems like an impossible feat to pen an adequate thank-you to the village of incredible people who made this book possible.

I have to start with the love of my life, Jesse, who has unwaveringly supported every single one of my crazy dreams over the last decade, no matter how big. Thank you for coming home after ten-hour shifts during a global pandemic and jumping in to scrub a mountain of dishes every night. For taste testing every recipe in this book and helping me make them better. And finally for serving endless cups of chamomile tea and pep talks as I sat crunched over my laptop during many late nights. You are simply the best.

I'm immensely grateful to my parents, Deb and Ken, and my sister, Jake, for inspiring my plant-based journey, love for amazing food, and the tenacity to always go after what I want. This book was no exception to the massive amount of support you have given me throughout my entire life. Thank you for recipe testing, editing, and talking me down from ledges every step of the way.

Wendy Sherman, my absolutely phenomenal agent, and her daughter Lexie for showing her my Instagram account. Thank you for taking a chance and sending me that fateful message in August 2019, asking if I've ever thought about writing a cookbook. None of this would exist without your faith in me, insight, encouragement, and support.

Renee Sedliar, my editor, to whom I am indebted. You brought my vision for *PlantYou* to life with your remarkable editing skills, constant positivity, and patience with me throughout the entire process. It was a dream come true to create this book with the entire brilliant team at Hachette Go, including Alison Dalafave, Cisca Schreefel, Laura Palese, Iris Bass, Katie Malm, Carrie Wicks, Elizabeth Parson, Zach Polendo, Ashley Kiedrowski, Michelle Aielli, and Michael Barrs.

Thank you to my multitalented best friend Stephanie McKnight of tidaldesign.ca, for beautifully editing the food photos you see in this book, shooting all the lifestyle images, and using her genius to develop the branding and logo for *PlantYou*.

Dr. Will Bulsiewicz, for encouraging me to write a cookbook, offering an endless amount of advice, and support on the process, and for penning a phenomenal foreword.

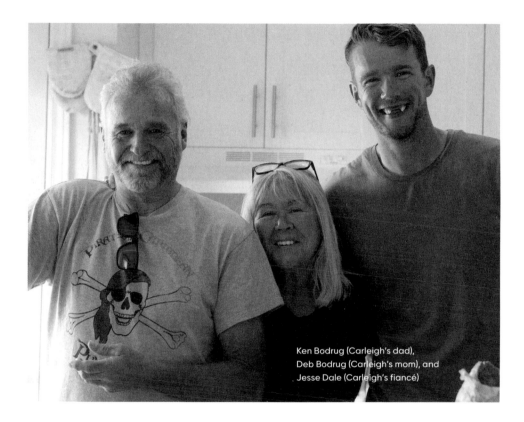

Ken Bodrug (Carleigh's dad),
Deb Bodrug (Carleigh's mom), and
Jesse Dale (Carleigh's fiancé)

Pam Kruusi and Cat Gavriusova for holding down the *PlantYou* fort while I wrote this cookbook without missing a single beat. I feel so lucky to have found two people who believe in the mission behind *PlantYou* as much as I do.

Thank you to all my dear friends and followers who tested the recipes and consulted on this book including Tracey Jakazi, Victoria Stacey, and Nicole Kraftscik.

My cat and companion, Tut. Thank you for keeping me company through lonely days of recipe testing and always humbling me with a disapproving glare.

And last, but certainly not least, thank you to the amazing *PlantYou* community. Your loyalty and support of my recipes over the years made it possible for me to bring this cookbook into the world. It is the honor of my life to be part of your plant-based journey.

Carleigh

endnotes

1   J. Poore and T. Nemecek. "Reducing Food's Environmental Impacts Through Producers and Consumers," *Science* 360, no. 6392 (2018), 987–992.

2   USDA Dietary Guidelines Advisory Committee, "Dietary Guidelines for Americans, 2010," 2010, https://www.fns.usda.gov/dietary-guidelines-previous-guidelines.

3   Dan Buettner, *The Blue Zones: 9 Lessons for Living Longer from the People Who've Lived the Longest* (Washington, DC: National Geographic Society, 2012).

4   Matt Zampa, "How Many Animals Are Killed for Food Every Day," Sentient Media, 2020, https://sentientmedia.org/how-many-animals-are-killed-for-food-every-day.

5   USDA, "Livestock, Dairy and Poultry Outlook," 2017, https://www.ers.usda.gov/webdocs /outlooks/86243/ldp-m-282.pdf.

6   Huffington Post, "9 Facts About Dairy Farming That Will Break Your Heart," 2014, https:// www.huffpost.com/entry/factory-farming-facts_n_4063892.

7   Chas Newkey-Burden, "Dairy Is Scary. The Public Are Waking Up to the Darkest Part of Farming," *Guardian*, 2017, https://www.theguardian.com/commentisfree/2017/mar/30 /dairy-scary-public-farming-calves-pens-alternatives.

8   Joel Fuhrman, "Olive Oil Is Not a Health Food," DrFuhrman.com, 2016, https://www .drfuhrman.com/elearning/eat-to-live-blog/84/olive-oil-is-not-a-health-food.

index

Note: Page references in *italics* indicate photographs.